SEXUAL PARTNERING, SEXUAL PRACTICES, AND HEALTH

SEXUAL PARTNERING, SEXUAL PRACTICES, AND HEALTH

Sana Loue, J.D., Ph.D., M.P.H.
Case Western Reserve University
Cleveland, Ohio

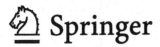 Springer

Sana Loue
Department of Epidemiology and Biostatistics
Case Western Reserve University
10900 Euclid Avenue
Cleveland, OH 44106-4945
USA
Sana.loue@case.edu

ISBN-10: 1-4899-9638-9
ISBN-13: 978-1-4899-9638-1
ISBN: 0-387-25986-4 (eBook)

Printed on acid-free paper.

9 8 7 6 5 4 3 2 1   SPIN 11396192

springeronline.com

We have been socialized to respect fear more than our own needs for language and definition, and while we wait in silence for that final luxury of fearlessness, the weight of that silence will choke us . . . . The transformation of silence into language and action is an act of self-revelation and that always seems fraught with danger . . . . We fear the very visibility without which we also cannot truly live . . . . And that visibility which makes us most vulnerable is also the source of our greatest triumph.

—Audre Lourde, 1977

[T]o speak a true word is to transform the world.

—Paolo Freire, 1978

Acknowledgements

This book would not have been possible without the research assistance of Nancy Mendez and Gary Edmunds.

Contents

Listing of Tables

Listing of Figures

Preface

Research tells us that sex is often "unsafe." A survey of sexual behavior reported that only 40% of 16 to 45 year olds in the U.K. consistently use a condom with a casual sex partner. This compares with 69% in France, 56% in the U.S., 48% in Italy, 36% in Spain, 32% in Germany, 28% in Russia, 25% in Canada, and 20% in Poland (Durex, 1996). Large proportions of individuals in the same age range say that they have been unfaithful in their relationships: 50% of Americans surveyed, 42% of British, 40% of Germans and Mexicans, 36% of French, and 22% of Spaniards (Durex, 1998). These figures portend the transmission of sexually transmitted infections, the possibility of pregnancy in the absence of contraception, and the physical and mental health consequences that may accompany chronic infection and/or unwanted or unplanned pregnancy. Monogamy has been touted as the proactive remedy for these unwanted consequences. Yet, it is assumed, first, that we all mean the same thing when we speak of monogamy and, second, that the structure of the relationship is determinative of both its quality and safety. However, sex may be unsafe for other reasons as well. "Partnering" may be accomplished through force, coercion, or outright violence. In such circumstances, the term "partnering" is a misnomer; there is no negotiation or mutuality in such situations.

Similarly, it has been asserted that two-parent households are more likely to have a positive effect on children than are other partnering arrangements. Such statements have ignored the context and quality of the partnering relationships to which the children may be exposed. It has been alleged that exposure to pornography will lead to increased aggressiveness. But, does the effect of viewing pornography vary between the individual who watches pornography online in the privacy or his or home and the individual who views it together with a group of beer-drinking buddies?

This book explores various dimensions of partnering, in an attempt both to re-contextualize sexual behavior within human exchanges and the social and political environments in which they exist, and to examine the health effects of various forms of partnering. Many of the ideas in this book are not new, but it is hoped that their re-visitation will prompt renewed efforts to examine behaviors in their context, rather than dissociated from the persons who perform them and the environments in which they occur.

Chapter 1 focuses on various understandings of monogamy or single pair-bonding between consenting adults. It becomes clear through this examination that, in discussing monogamy and the health implications of such an arrangement, that individuals may have very different conceptualizations of the topic under discussion. Chapter 2 examines family structures that consist of multiple adults as partners. Chapter 3 is concerned with "partnerings" that involve children: incest, pedophilia, and child marriage. In many such instances, if not the vast majority, the use of the word "partnering" is a misnomer because of the child's lack of ability to consent and/or the use of force or coercion to effectuate the sexual interaction. Chapter 4 addresses commercial partnering: sex work, trafficking, and pornography. Clearly, there is overlap between these concepts, just as there also exists interplay between child marriage and child trafficking, between pedophilia and child trafficking.

Chapter 5 explores object relations, that is, fetish behavior that is premised on an attraction to objects. Although chapter 5 is clearly delineated as having a focus on object relations, it must be kept in mind that, in many circumstances, such as commercial sex work and trafficking in humans for the purpose of sexual exploitation, the individuals involved in the encounter may view the other or be viewed as mere objects, rather than partners, in an exchange.

Each chapter concludes with a review of the health implications that flow from the partnerings examined. The final chapter discusses the implications of existing findings for research and practice.

CHAPTER 1

Diverse Monogamies

It was six men of Indostan
To learning much inclined,
Who went to see the Elephant
(Though all of them were blind),
That each by observation
Might satisfy his mind.

The First approached the Elephant,
And happening to fall
Against his broad and sturdy side,
At once began to bawl:
"God bless me! but the Elephant
Is very like a wall!"

The Second, feeling of the tusk,
Cried, "Ho! what have we here
So very round the smooth and sharp?
To me 'tis mighty clear
This wonder of an Elephant
Is very like a spear!"

The Third approached the animal,
And happening to take
The squirming trunk within his hands,
Thus boldly up and spake:

"I see," quoth he, "the Elephant
Is very like a snake!"

The Fourth reached out an eager hand,
And felt about the knee.
"What most this wondrous beast is like
Is mighty plain," quoth he;
"'Tis clear enough the Elephant
Is very like a tree!"

The Fifth, who chanced to touch the ear,
Said; "E'en the blindest man
Can tell what this resembles most;
Deny the fact who can,
This marvel of an Elephant
Is very like a fan!"

The Sixth no sooner had begun
About the beast to grope.
Than, seizing on the swinging tail
That fell within his scope,
"I see," quoth he, "the Elephant
Is very like a rope!"

And so these men of Indostand
Disputed loud and long,
Each in his own opinion
Exceeding stiff and strong,
Though each was partly in the right,
And all were in the wrong!

The Blind Men and the Elephant
John Godfrey Saxe

Defining Monogamy

Researchers reported from the National Health and Social Life Survey (NHSLS) that the vast majority of American men and women aged 18 to 59 are monogamous (Klitsch, 1995). Researchers have asserted that

most men and women in the world are monogamous (one spouse); they wed only one individual at a time. Many societies permit polygyny. But in most of these cultures only about 10 percent of men actually practice polygyny; even were polygyny is widespread, only about 25 percent of men have several wives at once. Monogamy is the hallmark of the human animal (Fisher, 1996).

Other researchers have presented contrary findings. One study concluded that, in a sample of 250 different cultures, 77% practiced some form of polygyny, 17% were monogamous, and 1% practiced polyandry (Murdock, 1967). Yet another review of data collected from 563 cultures from 6 regions of the world (Murdock, 1981) concluded that 78% of the cultures practiced polygyny, less than 1% practiced polyandry, and 21% were strictly monogamous (Altman and Ginat, 1996). Americans, in particular, have been accused of practicing non-monogamy, despite assertions of monogamy, by engaging in "serial monogamy" (cf. Frank, 2001). What, then, is monogamy?

Monogamy has been variously defined as

"the practice or state of being married to one person at a time" and is contrasted with 'polygamy,' defined as "having more than one wife or husband at the same time" (*Shorter Oxford English Dictionary*, quoted in Overall, 1998: 2)

the marriage of one man to one woman (Kanazawa and Still, 1999) a pattern by an individual of sexual interactions with only one other person during a given period within that individual's life, while "nonmonogamy" [means] a pattern by an individual of sexual interactions with more than one person during a given period within the individual's life (Overall, 1998: 4).

an exclusive sexual relationship between a woman and a man, whilst non-monogamy refers to a woman being involved in parallel, plural sexual relationships. Relationships can also be characterized by emotional or economic factors (Robinson, 1997).

fetishistic, for it makes a sexual fetish (not to mention a virtual possession) of one person exclusively . . . [M]onogamy, a form of marriage uniquely suited to capitalistic society, makes a fetish of persons and their bodies . . . a compromise between personal autonomy and interpersonal security which has survived in spite of itself. . . . (Smith and Smith, 1974: 33-35).

Yet other researchers have distinguished between "social monogamy" and sexual monogamy, arguing that, although U.S. culture assumes that social monogamy and sexual monogamy are synonymous, they aren't (Barash and Lipton, 2001; Hrdy, quoted in Morell, 1998). In contrast to sexual monogamy, social monogamy refers to the pairing up of individuals to live together, share resources, copulate, and produce and raise children. It has been asserted that "there is simply no question whether sexual desire for multiple partners is 'natural'. It is. Similarly, there is no question of monogamy being 'natural'. It isn't" (Barash and Lipton, 2001: 2). A similar dichotomy has been suggested by the distinction made between sexual exclusivity and possession and the creation of a long-term or life-long project with another person (Francis and Gontier, 1987). Accordingly, it has been argued, "aspiring monogamists are going against some of the deepest-seated evolutionary inclinations with which biology has endowed most creatures, *homo sapiens* included' (Barash and Lipton, 2001: 1).

Despite our apparent assumption that that we all mean the same thing when we use the term *monogamy*, there is clearly no consensus with respect to the definition of the term. As indicated by the above excerpts, the term monogamy has been used to refer to marital relationships only, sexual relationships only, male-female sexual relationships only, and a social-sexual dichotomy in relationships. The relevance and applicability of the concept to non-male-female relationships has also been challenged:

Lesbians and feminists continue to use words like *monogamy* and *non-monogamy* as if they made sense within a "feminist" conceptual framework when, in fact, they make *no sense*, especially when they're being used to describe Lesbian relationships! *Monogamy* means, literally, "marriage to one [woman]," and its contrastive term is *polygamy*, which means "marriage to more than one [woman]." I've added the term *woman*, in brackets, here because only men ever have the option of being married to more than one [woman]. These terms *assume* that women are the property of the men who marry them. Both *monogamy* and *nonmonogamy* name heteropatriarchal institutions within which the only important information is: *how many women can a man legitimately own?* Since the question of "ownership" is supposed to be a non-question in feminist and Lesbian-feminist relationships, I want to know *why* so many wimmin who claim to have a "raised consciousness" persist in using such words when they're supposed to know better? (Penelope, 1985: 35-36, italics in original).

Other difficulties, perhaps less evident, pervade our use of the term. The term monogamy conceives of a relationship, generally sexual, with one person at a time. Serial monogamy occurs when an exclusive relationship is terminated and is subsequently followed by another exclusive relationship (Robinson, 1997). As the time period between these exclusive relationships gradually diminishes, however, we must question whether the concept of monogamy is actually illusory.

Second, there is an underlying assumption, at least when speaking of U.S. culture, that monogamy equates to "fidelity," meaning that a failure to preserve sexual exclusivity within a relationship represents a breach of trust and, when that relationship is a marriage, constitutes adultery (Greeley, 1994; cf. Hite, 1991). This equation rests on the further assumption that all seemingly pair-bonded couples, regardless of the sex or sexual orientation of the partners, have similar notions regarding the exclusivity to be maintained within the framework of that relationship and that these notions are shared by both members of the couple. Such may not be the case. As an example, 1% of 1212 married adults participating in the General Social Survey indicated that sex with someone other than one's spouse while married is never wrong (Greeley, 1994). If, in fact, this opinion is reflective of the arrangement between the individuals in the marriage, it cannot be said to represent a breach of trust, thereby constituting "infidelity." Examined outside of the context of the relationship agreement, it has, however, been characterized by writers as such (Greeley, 1994).

Additionally, the term monogamy is most often contrasted with what is assumed to be its antonym, polygamy, thereby establishing an opposition between marriage to one individual and the simultaneous marriage to more than one individual. First, the use of each of these terms conceives of the relationship between the parties in the context of a legal or religious framework. Second, the contrast of one versus multiple marital partners fails to specify whether the expected exclusivity is sexual, social or both. The concept of romantic love thus appears dissociated from this dichotomy.

If, instead, monogamy is contrasted with non-monogamy, we find that the concept of monogamy is frequently associated with qualities of respect, trust, honesty, and love (Hite, 1991), while non-monogamy is said to be characterized by promiscuity, a shallowness of emotions, and a lack of commitment and security (Robinson, 1997). Indeed, non-monogamy is often equated with adultery, infidelity (Reibstein and Richards, 1992), "swinging," extramarital sex (Robinson, 1997), and the absence of emotional involvement and connection, despite evidence that some extramarital or extra-primary relationships may be of long duration and intense emotional connection (Sancton, 1996).

The inclusion of the term *polyamory* lends yet another dimension to this discussion and serves to underscore further the inadequacy of our language to describe simultaneously the multiple dimensions of relationships. Polyamory includes many different styles of multiple intimate involvements, such as polyfidelity or group marriage; primary relationships open to secondary affairs; and casual sexual involvement with two or more people (Munson and Stelboum, 1999: 2).

Other paradigms have been utilized in an attempt to characterize and distinguish between various types of sexual/romantic relationships. The term *cohabiting* has been used to refer to individuals who are living with their presumed partners, whether married or unmarried, sexually active with each other or not (Klitsch, 1995). The use of this term, like the use of the term monogamy, similarly implies, at least to some degree, a romantic or sexual connection between the individuals. These multiple dimensions and permutations of relationships are reflected in Figure 1, below.

Others have attempted to distinguish between the various types of relationships on the basis of the communication and exchange dynamics prevailing between the partners: the sentimental "romantic" relationship; the "hedonistic" relationship, entered into for passion and pleasure; the "matrimonial" relationship, characterized by feelings of security and concern for the other individual; and the "prostitutional" or utilitarian relationship, reflecting a system of exchange and an emphasis on individual goals (Ahlemeyer and Ludwig, 1997; Giami and Schiltz, 1996; Raj and Pollack, 1995). Still other researchers have delineated casual, secondary, and new relationships on the basis of their duration, exclusiveness, and investment in the long-term prospect of the relationship (Kordoutis, Loumakou, and Sarafidou, 2000).

In part, this lack of consensus may stem from varying perspectives of diverse disciplines, including biology, sociology, and psychology, to name but a few. To a great extent, however, we simply

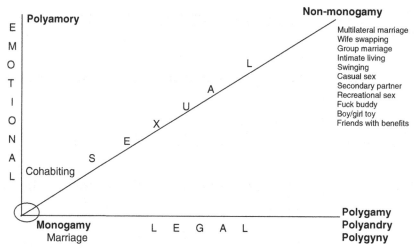

Figure 1. Dimensions of Partnered Relationships

lack language to comprehend the multiple levels, permutations, and types of relationships that can be entered into by two or more somehow-bonded adults. We can use the letters SA to denote Sexual Attachment, EA for Emotional Attachment, and LA for Legal Attachment and list the permutations of these dimensions that can occur with a relationship. It becomes more evident, then, that the complexities that are inherent in a relationship are not captured by the language that we use. As an example, $1(SA)=1(EA)$ would signify that an individual has one sexual attachment and one emotional attachment, and that the individual to whom he or she is sexually attached is the same individual to whom he or she is emotionally attached. In contrast, $(>1)SA \neq (>1)EA$ denotes the existence of multiple sexual attachments to individuals who are not the same as those with whom the individual has multiple emotional attachments.

$(1)SA=(1)EA$	$(1)LA=(1)SA \neq (1)EA$	$(>1)LA=(1)SA \neq (1)EA$
$(1)SA \neq (1)EA$	$(1)LA \neq (1)SA=(1)EA$	$(>1)LA \neq (1)SA=(1)EA$
$(>1)SA=(>1)EA$	$(1)LA \neq (1)SA \neq (1)EA$	$(>1)LA \neq (1)SA \neq (1)EA$
$(1)SA \neq (>1)EA$	$(1)LA \neq (>1)SA \neq (1)EA$	$(>1)LA=(>1)SA \neq (1)EA$

(>1)SA≠(1)EA   (1)LA≠(>1)SA=(>1)EA   (>1)LA=(>1)SA=(>1)EA

(>1)SA≠(>1)EA   (1)LA≠(>1)SA≠(>1)EA   (>1)LA≠(>1)SA=(>1)EA

(1)LA=(1)SA=(1)EA   (>1)LA=(1)SA=(1)EA   (>1)LA≠(>1)SA≠ (>1)EA

Origins of Pair-bonding/coupling

Multiple theories have been advanced to explain how and why pair-bonding/coupling, or monogamy as it is usually referred to, evolved. Researchers studying the evolution of mate partnerships among animals and birds have hypothesized that such partnerships represent an attempt to maximize the survival of the young: two parents were simply needed to assume the onerous burden of raising the young. It was assumed that males would do this only if the young were their own (Morell, 1998). However, in some species, such as bluebirds, although the male and female bond, build a nest, and raise chicks together, the female may have sexual encounters with other males and 15% to 20% of the chicks that are reared together may not have been sired by the partnering male (Black, 1996; Morell, 1998). More recently, experimental research involving prairie voles indicates that neuropeptide hormones released in the voles' brains may be associated with the formation of strong pair bonds (Morell, 1998).

Similar theories prevail with respect to the development of pair bonding in human populations. Not surprisingly, a biological basis has also been asserted for the maintenance, if not the initiation of, pair-bonding. Fisher has maintained that as we evolved, we developed the brain physiology for attachment (Frank, 1996). However, such attachments are required only long enough to rear a single child through its infancy, approximately four years. Subsequently, the pair may separate and form new pair bonds with new partners, potentially resulting in the production of varied offspring. Accordingly, Fisher has asserted, humans are not programmed for a life-long relationship but are, instead, biologically programmed for a series of relatively shorter ones. This biological programming does not, however, negate our ability to override our biological urges (Frank, 1996). Consistent with Fisher's premise, Marlowe (2000) has speculated that serial monogamy allows men with higher quality genes and higher status to achieve polygyny, or multiple pair bonding, as they age by allowing greater access to younger wives as they men age.

Herlihy (1995) maintains that the development of monogamy, that is, sexual and social pair-bonding between a male and a female, may have been either economically or socially imposed. The cooperation of one male and one female would have permitted the couple to exploit and defend the resources necessary to maintain themselves and their offspring. Monogamy became further entrenched due to the decline of slavery and the association of monogamy with morality by the Catholic church (Herlihy, 1995), effectuated through the cessation of concubinage by elite males and through the establishment of prohibitions against divorce and endogamous marriages and penalties for illegitimacy (MacDonald, 2001). Once established, monogamy served as a stabilizing force (Herlihy, 1995).

Alexander (1987) and colleagues (Alexander, Hoogland, Howard, Noonan, and Sherman, 1979) have also speculated that monogamy developed due to environmental and/or social conditions. Ecologically imposed monogamy was said to result from environmental conditions that rendered it impossible for men to "gain by attempting to provide for offspring of more than one wife" (Alexander, Hoogland, Howard, Noonan, and Sherman, 1979: 418-419). Socially imposed monogamy resulted from the imposition of laws designed to prohibit polygyny and promote or prescribe monogamy (Alexander, 1987).

Monogamy has also been said to represent, at least in part, a compromise or concession made by upper-class men to lower-class men in exchange for their political support (Alexander, 1987;

Alexander, Hoogland, Howard, Noonan, and Sherman, 1979; Betzig, 1986; MacDonald, 1990). Hawkes' theory is not inconsistent: that monogamy arose as the result of negotiations between males about access to females, in an attempt to reduce the risks inherent in direct fighting between competing men (Hagmann, 1999).

In contrast to these theories, Kanazawa and Still (1999) maintain that the institution of marriage, which they equate with monogamy, emerged due to the gradual decline of inequality among men and women's conscious choice to marry monogamously rather than polygynously. Sanderson (2001) has pointed out the fallacy underlying this theory, noting that polygyny appears to result from male, rather than female, choice due to a male desire for sexual variety, which presumably evolved in order to promote male reproductive success.

Feminist writers have focused on the social and cultural factors that have encouraged the development of pair-bonded relationships. Rosa asserts

that monogamy is enforced by cultural products (the media), economic restraints (tax incentives, the high cost of single living), social factors (the provision of support and companionship, or social status and privilege) and by the notion that this is "how it is", "this is natural" (Rosa, 1994: 108).

Others have argued that the idealization of monogamy has been used to control women (Tsoulis, 1987).

Monogamy and Health

Monogamy, Safer Sex, and Infectious Disease

Public health advisories stress the importance of monogamous relationships and protective strategies, such as condom use, as mechanisms to reduce the risk of transmission of diseases such as HIV/AIDS, syphilis, gonorrhea, and Chlamydia. One must logically ask, What are the consequences of a failure to utilize safer sex precautions, such as monogamy or condoms? It has been estimated that a woman engaging in 50 unprotected acts of vaginal intercourse with 50 different sexual partners has a 55% chance of pregnancy, a 5% chance of contracting Chlamydia, and a .001% chance of contracting HIV in a U.S. low-risk population (Cohen and Bruce, 1997). The HIV risk increases to .002% in the college population.

As indicated, longer term relationships, cohabiting relationships, and "steady" relationships are often presumed by at least one of the participating partners to be monogamous when such may not be the case. A review of 12 surveys conducted between 1948 and 1981 found that the proportion of men reporting extramarital sex ranged from 20% to 66% of the samples, while 10% to 69% of the samples of female participants reported having had extramarital sex (Thomson, 1983). Later studies reported that an average of 72% of men married for 2 or more years acknowledged having had extramarital sex (Hite, 1981), and 70% of women who had been married for more than 5 years had engaged in extramarital relations (Hite, 1987).

The 1991 General Social Survey of 1212 individuals conducted by the National Opinion Research Center found that 11% of the female respondents and 21% of the participating males indicated having had sexual relations with someone other than their spouse during their marriage (Greeley, 1994). Among men, sex outside of marriage was associated with a belief that adultery is not wrong, dissatisfaction with family life, a perception of poor health, recent psychological counseling, and self-reported drunkenness and smoking. Among women, predictors of extramarital sex included loss of a job, conflict with a spouse, trouble with a child, dissatisfaction with family life, and psychological counseling. In general, sex outside of marriage among women was more frequently associated with difficulties in a relationship (spouse, child, or family) as compared with men having sex outside of marriage.

Sexual relations outside of cohabiting, nonmarried living arrangements also appear common. Results of the British National Survey of Sexual Attitudes and Lifestyles indicate that over a 5-year period, almost two-third of the men and just under one-half of the women reported having more than one sexual partner during the previous year (Johnson, Wadsworth, Wellings, and Field, 1994). In this same study, only 21.8% of the married women and 26.2% of the unmarried, cohabiting women used condoms for contraception, placing them at potential risk of infection with a sexually transmitted disease.

Research has found that men hold varying beliefs about monogamy. A survey of 486 men yielded several major themes relating to monogamy: monogamy would help to build trust and respect from their partner, demonstrate love, provide protection from HIV and STDs, signify the ability to satisfy their partner, and represent a loss of opportunities to have sexual relations with other women (Gillmore, Stielstra, Huang, Baker, Beadnell, and Morrison, 2003). Compared to unmarried men, men who were married and living with their wives exhibited more favorable attitudes towards monogamy.

African-American women with a strong sense of ethnic identity have been found to have more favorable normative beliefs about monogamy (Beadnell, Stielstra, Baker, Morrison, Knox, Gutierrez, and Doyle, 2003). It has been hypothesized that ethnic identity, reflecting a sense of belonging to one's ethnic group and a positive evaluation of the group, enhances self-esteem and social support, thereby leading to greater individual self-protection (Belgrave, Van Oss Marin, and Chambers, 2000; Brook, Balka, Brook, Win, and Gursen, 1988; Brook, Whieman, Balka, Win, and Gursen, 1988).

Research indicates that individuals in extended relationships are more likely to discuss their sexual histories than are individuals practicing serial monogamy, while those engaging in casual sexual encounters have been found least likely to discuss their sexual histories (Cohen and Bruce, 1997).

Numerous studies have found that individuals are more likely to use condoms with casual partners than they are with their primary relationship partners. A review of studies focusing on relationships statuses and the practice of safer sex identified 54 studies that found condom use less frequent with established relationship, cohabiting, or primary partners than with casual/one-might stand, nonrelationship, anonymous, and commercial partners (Misovich, Fisher, and Fisher, 1997). A qualitative study with 23 women over the age of 30 found that condom usage appeared more problematic in longer term relationships as compared with more casual relationships (Maxwell and Boyle, 1995). Many of the women indicated that they were not at risk because they were in long term relationships, despite their acknowledgement that the long term relationship had not been monogamous due to their partner's behavior. Other study participants found it difficult to initiate safer sex with condoms after learning of their partners' extra-relationship sexual behaviors because they had not previously used condoms. Findings from the 1998 Canadian Contraception Study similarly found that a large proportion of women believed that having only one sexual partner obviated the need to utilize measures to reduce HIV risk (29%) and that once a woman knew and trusted her partner, condoms would no longer be needed for STD/AIDS prevention (26%)(Fisher, Boroditsky, and Bridges, 1999).

Accordingly, it has been hypothesized that the trust and security of a long-term relationship may not only foster attraction and intimacy, but may also foster a belief that the partner is safe and lessen motivation to use HIV knowledge (Clark, 1994a, 1994b). It has been suggested that individuals may have consistently unprotected sex in multiple relationships due to biases in perceiving relationships in general. Serial monogamy could be used to illustrate the point. Perhaps individuals should learn how to maintain focus on safe sex practices against competing subjective representations of relationships that misleadingly confound safe sex with quality features of the relationship (Kordoutis, Loumakou, and Sarafidou, 2000).

Child Development

Research relating to child development has tended to focus on the structure of the partner relationship, rather than on its dynamic or quality. This focus is premised on a belief that knowledge of children's functioning in different family structures will inform social policy, which can then be framed to maximize the well-being of future generations (Garfinkel and McLanahan, 1990; Seltzer, 1994). Consequently, available studies often compare child development in the context of a two-parent (married or cohabiting) family with child development in a single-parent or multi-parent family. This section focuses on child development in families that would be characterized as single or dual parent. Child development in the context of multi-parent families will be addressed in Chapter 2.

Study findings from various national surveys indicate that children raised in two-parent households do better in measures of educational achievement and adjustment than those raised in single parent households, the majority of which are headed by single mothers. It has been asserted that children raised in two-parent households have an advantage due to an increased socioeconomic level and because single mothers have less social support, poorer psychological well-being, and lower educational levels (Carlson and Corcoran, 2001; Dunn, Deater-Deckard, Pickering, and O'Connor, 1998; McLanahan and Sandefur, 1994; O'Connor, Dunn, Jenkins, Pickering, and Rabash, 2001).

Observations such as these have prompted concerns that children in single-parent families may experience relatively fewer social relationships with nonmaternal adults, resulting in serious deficits in interpersonal resources in comparison with children of two-parent families (Amato, 1995). It has been asserted that children of single parents will have fewer positive, warm interactions with adults, will lack adult male role models (Cochran, Larner, Riley, Gunnarsson, and Henderson, 1990; McLanahan and Booth, 1989; McLanahan and Bumpass, 1988), and will be subject to less discipline and supervision (Dornbusch, Carlsmith, Bushwall et al., 1985; Dornbusch, Ritter, Leiderman, Roberts, and Farleigh, 1987; Steinberg, 1987), resulting in relatively poorer emotional, behavioral, and cognitive functioning. These fears have been exacerbated by recent data indicating that nearly one-quarter of children in recent birth cohorts will spend at least some time in single-parent households due to divorce, and another quarter will reside with a single mother due to non-marital childbearing (Bumpass and Raley, 1993).

These fears have prompted policymakers at various levels of government to formulate pro-marriage policies. President George W. Bush stated at the Fourth National Summit on Fatherhood on June 7, 2001: "If we are serious about renewing fatherhood, we must be serious about renewing marriage." Accordingly, federal welfare reforms have eliminated disincentives to marriage; established programs to promote marriage; and provided incentives, such as cash rewards, to couple who marry (Brito, 2002). The state of West Virginia, with the approval of the federal Department of Health and Human Services, pays an additional $100 per month to families in which the parents are married and residing together and are both named on the check. These policies reflect the perspective of David Popenoe, director of the Rutgers Marriage Project, who testified before the Subcommittee on Human Resources of the U.S. House of Representatives:

Left culturally unregulated, men's sexual behavior can be promiscuous, their paternity casual, their commitment to families weak. Marriage is society's way of engaging the basic problem of fatherhood—how to hold the father to the stronger mother-child bond (May 22, 2001. Quoted in Jaffee, Moffitt, Caspi, and Taylor, 2003: 110).

As in research and policy statements relating to monogamy or multi-partnering, the single-faceted depictions of families as single- or dual-parent and the formulations of policies such as these ignore the complexities that characterize the relationship and environmental contexts in favor of a simplistic analysis and resolution. Research findings negate the wisdom of this approach.

First, research data indicate that the characterization of families as single- or dual-parent assumes a homogeneity of structure across families that may not exist. The label of "single-parent family" may include not only families headed by a single biological parent, but also those that are comprised of a single parent (mother or father) and extended family. Dual-parent families may reflect a variety of constellations, including two married biological parents; one biological parent and a stepparent to whom he or she is married; one biological parent and a cohabiting, nonmarital sexual partner; one biological parent and a cohabiting, nonmarital, nonsexual partner; and two nonbiological adults, married or cohabiting, who may be serving as parents, such as in the case of adoptive or foster parents. Yet a third alternative, not reflected in comparisons of single-parent and dual-parent families, is that of a family comprised of extended members only, such as grandparents, uncle and aunts, cousins, etc. Research and clinical practice that rests on a family deficit model, which presupposes that children living in single-parent families where the father is absent will experience poorer psychosocial and behavioral outcomes than children from "intact", i.e. dual-parent, families (Partridge and Kotler, 1987), fail to recognize this diversity in structure.

Second, regardless of how a family is constituted or self-defines, there is significant heterogeneity in functioning across families. Families differ in their approaches to discipline, the degree of parental control and child compliance, the looseness of the family structure, the degree to which children function autonomously, and the management of conflict (Florsheim, Tolan, and Gorman-Smith, 1998).

Third, investigations of family structure alone as a determinative factor on child development fail to consider the heterogeneity of fathers, father-child relationships, mothers, and mother-child relationships. Data from the Fragile Families Study, which followed a birth cohort of 4700 U.S. schoolchildren, indicate that, compared with married fathers, unwed fathers were more likely to have been under the age of 20 at the time of the interview, to have lower levels of education and lower incomes, to have used illicit drugs several times a month, to have engaged in partner violence, and to have reported moderate to high levels of depression (Wilson and Brooks-Gunn, 2001). Several other studies have similarly found that men who had children before marriage have lower levels of educational achievement, lower incomes, and higher levels of unemployment (Jaffee, Caspi, Moffitt, Taylor, and Dickson, 2001; Nock, 1998). In addition, they may be more likely to experience symptoms of anxiety, to suffer from drug and alcohol problems, and to engage in crime, violence, and abuse of women (Jaffee, Caspi. Moffitt, Taylor, and Dickson, 2001). Yet other research reports that fathers' antisocial behavior may increase children's risk for conduct problems (Jaffee, Moffitt, Casper, and Taylor, 2003) due to family poverty (Moffitt and the E-Risk Study Team, 2002), child and spousal abuse (Farmington, 1994; Margolin and Gordis, 2000), harsh and coercive discipline (Fagot, Pears, Capaldi, Crosby, and Leve, 1998), and comorbid drug and alcohol problems (Robins, 1998). Accordingly, it is critical that research and practice consider the quality of a father's presence, and not merely the fact of his presence or absence.

Similarly, research findings suggest that it is the quality of the mother-child relationship, rather than the fact of single- or dual-parenting, that may be critical to a child's development. It has been found, for instance, that children in single mother families received more support than children living in other family constellations due to increased social support available to the mothers, increased diligence by the mothers to compensate for the fathers' absence, and/or the support of youth by their absent fathers or other male role models (Zimmerman, Salem, and Maton, 1995).

Finally, a focus on family structure alone fails to acknowledge the multiplicity and interrelatedness of factors that contribute to child development. As an example, income level and child gender have been found to be the strongest predictors of children's conduct and peer relations, rather than family composition (Patterson, Kupersmidt, and Vaden, 1990).

Implications for Research and Practice

This chapter has presented an overview of the concepts of various partner configurations, including monogamy, polygyny, polyandry, polygamy, and polyamory. It is clear from this review that our language, including our use of these terms, inadequately reflects the multidimensional, multifaceted nature of various partner configurations.

Unfortunately, this imprecision extends to our research. Research may be founded on underlying assumptions that may not apply to the population under examination, yet the researchers may be unaware that they are doing so. As an example, surveys of people's sexual behavior may fail to make clear exactly what is meant by the use of terms such as "monogamy," assuming that everyone has the same definition of the term. Such assumptions magnify the initial imprecision of the language that we use, potentially resulting in unreliable or invalid conclusions.

The conclusions that we draw from research may also suffer due to a failure to contextualize our research questions and our findings. As an example, many studies of child development classify families on the basis of single- or dual-parents in the household. This uni-dimensional characterization fails to consider the larger context in which the families function, the nature and quality of any partner relationship that the parent(s) may have, the nature and quality of the adult-child relationships that exist for a particular child, and the multiplicity of factors that impact a child's development.

The erroneous inferences that are drawn from research as a result of unrecognized and unacknowledged imprecision and assumptions may negatively, but unknowingly, affect the ability of clinicians to address the needs of their patients or clients. Physicians and other health practitioners may assume that the patient need not be counseled about the prevention of sexually transmitted infections, based on the patient's representations that he or she is in a long-term monogamous relationship. This approach may be ill-advised, due to varying conceptualizations of monogamy and the possibility that the patient's partner may be engaging in other sexual relations that are unknown to the patient. Social workers and other counselors may assume that the behavior problems of the adolescent son of a relatively poor single mother are due to the absence of a father figure and adequate family income when, in fact, the child may have multiple positive male role models in the family network.

References

Ahlemeyer, H.W., Ludwig, D. (1997). Norms of communication and communication as norm in the intimate social system. In L. van Campenhoudt, M. Cohen, G. Guizzardi, D. Hausser (Eds.). *Sexual Interactions and HIV Risk: New Conceptual Perspectives in European Research* (pp. 142-159). London: Taylor and Francis.

Alexander, R.D. (1987). *The Biology of Moral Systems*. Hawthorne: Aldine de Gruyter.

Alexander, R.D., Hoogland, J.L., Howard, R.D., Noonan, K.M., Sherman, P.W. (1979). Sexual dimorphisms and breeding systems in pinnipeds, ungulates, primates, and humans. In N.A. Chagnon, W. Irons (Eds.). *Evolutionary Biology and Human Social Behavior* (pp. 402-435). North Scituate, Massachusetts: Duxbury Press.

Altman, I., Ginat, J. (1996). *Polygamous Families in Contemporary Society*. Cambridge, U.K.: Cambridge University Press.

Amato, P.R. (1995). Single-parent households as settings for children's development, well-being, and attainment: A social network/resources perspective. *Sociological Studies of Children* 7: 19-47.

Barash, D.P., Lipton, J.E. (2001). *The Myth of Monogamy: Fidelity and Infidelity in Animals and People*. New York: W.H. Freeman and Company.

Betzig, L. (1986). *Despotism and Differential Reproduction: A Darwinian View of History*. New York: Aldine.

Black, J.M. (1996). *The Study of Monogamy*. New York: Oxford University Press.

Brito, T.L. (2002). I'll Take Bachelor Number One!: The Promotion of Marriage as an Anti-Poverty Policy. Unpublished manuscript, University of Wisconsin, Madison, Wisconsin. Cited in S.R. Jaffee, T.E. Moffitt, A. Caspi, A. Taylor. (2003). Life with (or without) father: The benefits of living with two biological parents depends on the father's antisocial behavior. *Child Development* 74(1): 109-126.

Bumpass, L.L., Raley, K.K. (1993). Trends in the duration of single-parent families. National Survey of Families and Households. Working Paper No. 58, Center for Demography and Ecology, University of Wisconsin, Madison, Wisconsin. Cited in J.A. Seltzer. (1994). Consequences of marital dissolution for children. *Annual Review of Sociology* 20: 235-266.

Carlson, M.J., Corcoran, M.E. (2001). Family structure and children's behavioral and cognitive outcomes. *Journal of Marriage and the Family* 63: 779-792.

Carroll, L. (1991). Gender, knowledge about AIDS, reported behavioral change, and the sexual behavior of college students. *Journal of American College Health* 40: 5-12.

Clark, L.F. (1994a). Partner perceptions, HIV risk behaviors, and risk-reduction behaviors. Paper presented at meeting of Society of Experimental Social Psychology, Lake Tahoe, California.

Clark, L.F. (1994b). Perceived safety in partner choice. Paper presented at meeting of the American Psychological Association, Los Angeles, California.

Cochran, M., Larner, M., Riley, D., Gunnarsson, L., Henderson, C.R. (1990). *Extending Families: The Social Networks of Parents and Their Children.* New York: Cambridge University Press.

Cohen, D.J., Bruce, K.E. (1997). Sex and mortality: Real risk and perceived vulnerability. *Journal of Sex Research* 34(3): 279-191.

Dornbusch, S.M., Carlsmith, J.M., Bushwall, S.J., Ritter, P.L., Leiderman, H., Hastorf, A.H., Gross, R.T. (1985). Single parents, extended households, and the control of adolescents. *Child Development* 56: 326-341.

Dornbusch, S.M., Ritter, P.L., Leiderman, P.H., Roberts, D.F., Farleigh, M.J. (1987). The relation of parenting style to adolescent school performance. *Child Development* 48: 1244-1257.

Du Bois, B. (1983). Passionate scholarship: Notes on values, knowing and method in feminist social science. In G. Bowles, R.D. Klein (Eds.). *Theories of Women's Studies.* London: Routledge & Kegan Paul.

Dunn, J., Deater-Deckard, K., Pickering, K., O'Connor, T.G. (1998). Children's adjustment and prosocial behaviour in step-, single-parent, and non-stepfamily settings: Findings from a community study. *Journal of Child Psychology and Psychiatry* 39: 1083-1095.

Florsheim, P., To Lan, P., Gorman-Smith, D. (1998). Family relationships, parenting practices, the availability of male family members, and the behavior of inner-city boys in single-mother and two-parent families. *Child Development* 69: 1437-1447.

Fagot, B.I., Pears, K.C., Capaldi, D.M., Crosby, L., & Leve, C.S. (1998). Becoming and adolescent father: Precursors and parenting. *Developmental Psychology* 34: 1209-1219.

Farrington, D.P. (1994). Childhood, adolescent and adult features of violent males. In L.R. Huesmann (Ed.), *Aggressive Behavior: Current Perspectives* (pp. 215-240). New York: Plenum.

Francis, C., Gontier, F. (1987). *Simone de Beauvoir: A Life . . . A Love Story.* (Trans. L. Nesselson). New York: St. Martin's.

Frank, C. (2001). Why do we fall in—and out of—love? Dr. Helen Fisher unravels the mystery. *Biography Magazine* February: 95-97, 112.

Garfinkel, I., McLanahan, S.S. (1990). The effects of child support provisions of the Family Support Act of 1988 on child well-being. *Population Research and Policy Review* 9: 205-234.

Giami, A., Schiltz, M.A. (1996). Representations of sexuality and relations between partners: Sex research in France in the era of AIDS. *Annual Review of Sex Research* 7: 125-157.

Greeley, A. (1994). *Society* 31(4): 9-13.

Haggman, M. (1999). More questions about the provider's role. *Science* 283(5403): 777-779.

Herlihy, D. (1995). Biology and history: The triumph of monogamy. *Journal of Interdisciplinary History* 25(4): 571-583.

Hite, S. (1991). *The Hite Report on Love, Passion and Emotional Violence.* London: Optima.

Hite, S. (1981). *The Hite Report on Male Sexuality.* London: Macdonald Optima.

Hite, S. (1987). *The Hite Report: Women and Love: A Cultural Revolution in Progress.* London: Penguin Books Ltd.

Jaffee, S.R., Caspi, A., Moffitt, T.E., Taylor, A., Dickson, N. (2001). Predicting early fatherhood and whether young fathers live with their children: Prospective findings and policy reconsiderations. *Journal of Child Psychology and Psychiatry* 42: 803-815.

Jaffee, S.R., Moffitt, T.E., Caspi, A., Taylor, A. (2003). Life with (or without) father: The benefits of living with two biological parents depends on the father's antisocial behavior. *Child Development* 74(1): 109-126

Johnson, A.M., Wadsworth, J., Wellings, K., Field, J. (1994). *Sexual Attitudes and Lifestyles.* Oxford, England: Blackwell Scientific Publications.

Kanazawa, S. Still, M.C. (1999). Why monogamy? *Social Forces* 78(1): 25-50.

Klitsch, M. (1995). Monogamy is the rule, many partners are the exception among most Americans, first U.S. sex survey finds. *Family Planning Perspectives* 27(1): 37-39.

Kordoutis, P.S., Loumakou, M., Sarafidou, J.O. (2000). Heterosexual relationship characteristics, condom use, and safe sex practices. *AIDS Care* 12(6): 767-782.

MacDonald, K. (1990). Mechanisms of sexual egalitarianism in Western Europe. *Ethology and Sociobiology* 11: 195-238.

MacDonald, K. (2001). Theoretical pluralism and historical complexity in the development and maintenance of socially imposed monogamy: A comment on Kanazawa and Still. *Social Forces* 80(1): 343-347.

Margolin, G., Gordis, E.B. (2000). The effects of family and community violence on children. *Annual Review of Psychology* 51: 445-479.

Marlowe, F. (2000). The patriarchal hypothesis: An alternative explanation of menopause. *Human Nature* 11: 27-42.

Maxwell, C., Boyle, M. (1995). Risky heterosexual practices amongst women over 30: Gender, power and long term relationships. *AIDS Care* 7(3): 277-294.

McLanahan, S., Booth, K. (1989). Mother-only families: Problems, prospects, and politics. *Journal of Marriage and the Family* 51: 557-580.

McLanahan, S., Bumpass, L. (1988). Intergenerational consequences of family disruption. *American Journal of Sociology* 1: 130-152.

McLanahan, S., Sandefur, G. (1994). *Growing Up with a Single Parent: What Hurts, What Helps.* Cambridge, Massachusetts: Harvard University Press.

Moffitt, T.E., E-Risk Study Team. (2002). Teen-aged mothers in contemporary Britain. *Journal of Child Psychology and Psychiatry* 43: 727-742.

Morell, V. (1998). A new look at monogamy. *Science* 281 (5385): 1982-1983.

Munson, M., Stelboum J. (1999). Introduction. In M. Munson, J.P. Stelboum (Eds.). *The Lesbian Polyamory Reader: Open Relationships,*

Non-Monogamy, and Casual Sex (pp. 1-7). New York: Haworth Press, Inc.

Murdock, G.P. (1981). *Atlas of World Cultures*. Pittsburgh, Pennsylvania: University of Pittsburgh Press.

Murdock, G.P. (1967). *Social Structure*. New York: Macmillan.

Nock, S.L. (1998). The consequences of premarital fatherhood. *American Sociological Review* 63: 250-263.

O'Connor, T.G., Dunn, J., Jenkins, J., Pickering, K., Rabash, J. (2001). Family settings and children's adjustment: Differential adjustment within and across families. *British Journal of Psychiatry* 179: 110-115.

Overall, C. (1998). Monogamy, nonmonogamy, and identity. *Hypatia* 13(4): 1-17.

Partridge, S., Kotler, T. (1987). Self-esteem and adjustments in adolescents from bereaved, divorced and intact families: Family type versus family environment. *Australian Journal of Psychology* 39: 223-234.

Patterson, C.J., Kupersmidt, J.B., Vaden, N.A. (1990). Income level, gender, ethnicity, and household composition as predictors of children's school-based competence. Child development 61: 485-494.

Penelope, J. (1985). The mystery of lesbians. *Lesbian Ethics* 1(2): 79-105.

Qulliam, S. (1994). *Women on Sex*. London: Smith Gryphon.

Raj, A.J., Pollack, R.H. (1995). Factors predicting high risk sexual behavior in heterosexual college students. *Journal of Sex and Marital Therapy* 21: 213-224.

Reibstein, J., Richard, M. (1992). *Sexual Arrangements: Marriage, Monogamy and Affairs*. London: William Heineman.

Robins, L.N. (1998). The intimate connection between antisocial personality and substance abuse. *Social Psychiatry and Psychiatric Epidemiology* 33: 393-399.

Robinson, V. (1997). My baby just cares for me: Feminism, heterosexuality, and non-monogamy. *Journal of Gender Studies* 6(2): 143-157.

Rosa, B. (1994). Anti-monogamy: A challenge to compulsory heterosexuality. In G. Griffin, M. Hester, S. Raj, S. Roseneil (Eds.). *Stirring It, Challenges for Feminism*. London: Taylor and Francis.

Sancton, T. (1996) Adieu, Mitterand. *Time Europe*, January 22. Available at http://www.Time.com/time/Europe/timetrails/france/france960122.html.
Last accessed March 29, 2005.

Sanderson, S.K. (2001). Explaining monogamy and polygyny in human societies: Comment on Kanazawa and Still. *Social Forces* 80(1): 329-336.

Smith, J.R., Smith, L.G. (1974). *Beyond Monogamy: Recent Studies of Sexual Alternatives in Marriage.* Baltimore, Maryland: Johns Hopkins Press.

Steinberg, L. (1987). Single parents, stepparents, and the susceptibility of adolescents to antisocial peer pressure. *Child Development* 58: 269-275.

Thompson, A.P. (1983). Extramarital sex: A review of the research literature. *Journal of Sex Research* 19: 1-22.

Tsoulis, A. (1987). Heterosexuality—a feminist option. *Spare Rib* June(179): 22-26.

Wilson, M., Brooks-Gunn, J. (2001). The health status and behaviors of unwed fathers. *Children and Youth Services Review* 23: 377-401.

Zimmerman, M.A., Salem, D.A., Maton, K.I. (1995). Family structure and psychosocial correlates among urban African-American adolescent males. *Child Development* 66: 1598-1613.

CHAPTER 2

Multi-Bonding: Polygamy, Polygyny, Polyamory

Defining and Identifying Multi-bonding

Non-monogamous relationships can take any number of forms, including, but not limited to, serial pair-bonding (known most frequently as serial monogamy), polygamy, polyandry, communal living, and "open" pair-bondings, where sexual or sexual-emotional relationships outside of the primary one are tolerated to a greater or lesser degree (cf. Robinson, 1997). *Polygyny* has been defined as "the marriage of a man to two or more women at the same time" (Moorehead, 1991: 311), or the "practice of plural marriage" (Altman and Ginat, 1996: 3). The term *polygamy* has also been used synonymously with polygyny, although it could also be used to encompass polyandry (Welch and Glick, 1981). *Polyandry* refers to the marriage of one woman to two or more husbands, while *polygynandry* contemplates a situation in which two or more women are simultaneously married to two or more men (Al-Krenawi, Graham, and Slonim-Nevo, 2002). *Polygynandry* has also been used to refer to group marriage (Anon., 2004). The term *informal polygamy* has been used to describe relationships characterized by the simultaneous existence of a legal marriage of one man to one woman and an affair with a second woman that has become a stable feature of the family structure (Rivett and Street, 1993). In contrast, *polyamory* refers to "group marriage" or the existence of one or more sexual

27

relationships inside or outside of marriage (Munson and Stelboum, 1999).

The incidence of polygamy, used here to refer to bonded relationships between one man and multiple women or one woman and multiple men entered into in a legal or religious context, has been shown to vary across cultures. Researchers have found that in Africa, the incidence of polygamy tends to be higher in the West and less in other regions of the continent (Lesthaeghe, Kaufmann, and Meekers, 1987) and is considered a valid form of marriage in Algeria, Benin, Chad, Congo, Ghana, Togo, Tanzania (Welch and Glick, 1981), Saudi Arabia, and among the Bedouin-Arab communities of Israel. As of 1975, almost one-half of all marriages in Ibadan, Nigeria were thought to be polygamous (Ware, 1979). It has been estimated that anywhere from one-fifth to one-half of all marriages in Africa are polygamous (Caldwell and Caldwell, 1993). The incidence of polygamy among men in Zaire was estimated in 1977 to be approximately 29.8% (Pitshandege, 1978, cited in Welch III and Glick, 1981). According to the 1966 census, approximately 46,854 of 4,830,316 men in Iran, or slightly less than 1%, had multiple wives (Momeni, 1975), whereas it has been estimated that in Kuwait, between 8% and 13% of all marriages are polygamous. According to estimates derived at various points in time from 1957 through 1964, for every 1,000 men, 220 in Chad, 320 in Upper Volta, 290 in Cameroon, and 230 in Mali were in polygamous marriages (Tabutin, 1974). The percentage of younger women (ages 20 to 29) involved in polygynous unions has been found to vary widely across African nations, from 8% in Lesotho to 35% in Senegal (Lauras-Lecoh, 1990).

Origins of Multi-bonding

Numerous factors have been identified that appear to influence the occurrence of multi-bonding in human populations. (For a relatively brief discussion of its evolution in bird and animal species, the reader is urged to consult Grønstøl, Byrkjedal, and Fiksen, 2003; Ptak and Lachmann, 2003). The demographic perspective posits that males may experience higher rates of mortality than females due to disease, warfare, and/or occupational dangers associated with activities such as hunting, ocean fishing, and migration labor (Dorjahn, 1959). This elevated rate of male mortality may be responsible, at least in part, for an increase in polygyny (Lee, 1979). Polygyny may also be attributable to warfare because of the resultant high rates of male mortality (Murdock, 1949) and the ability of the conquering men to capture women from the vanquished opponents (Dorjahn, 1959).

A study of the Ngwa Igbo in Nigeria identified five principal reasons for men to maintain more than one wife: because having more than one wife allows the Ngwa husband to (1) have the many children that he desires; (2) heighten his prestige and boost his ego among his peers; (3) enhance his status within his community; (4) ensure a sufficient availability of labor to perform the necessary farm work and the processing of commercial oil-palm produce; and (5) satisfy his sexual urges (Uchendu, 1965). Indian Muslim men have offered various reasons for having taken additional wives: to have a better life-partner, to be able to have a child because the first wife is barren, to ameliorate the lack of "homeness" in their homes resulting from the primary wife's long-term illness, to restore "light and laughter" to their lives, to increase the household income through the additional wife's wages from employment, and to reduce their level of frustration with the first wife that resulted from her lack of consideration and temperament (Haqqi, 1974).

A need for alliances between families and clans has also served as a motivating force behind a polygamous marriages (Hillman, 1975). As an example, "exchange marriages" have been found to be common in Bedouin-Arab communities, whereby two males marry each other's sisters. If one of the husbands takes a second wife, the other husband may feel pressured to do the same (Al-Krenawi and Graham 1999).

Religious belief also appears to play a role in the formation of formalized polygynous unions. As an example, 92% of the population of Mali identifies as Muslim (Madhavan, 2002). Islam permits men to have as many as four wives (El Azayem and Hedayat-Diba, 1994; Madhavan, 2002) and views polygamy as protecting the family from possible deviation to illegal sexual intercourse and from contracting sexually transmitted diseases (El Azayem and Hedayat-Diba, 1994). Consequently, it is not surprising that 45% of Mali's married women have been found to be in polygynous unions (Madhavan, 2002). In Ghana, polygamous marriages have been found to be more frequent among Muslim women who ascribe to traditional religious beliefs (Klomegah, 1997). However, a study of polygamy among Muslims in India found that a minority were in polygamous marriages (Haqqi, 1974).

Although much of what we know about multi-bonding comes to us from studies of various groups and societies in Africa (see below), the issue of multi-bonding is relevant in the United States today, despite the illegality of formal, legalized multiple unions. First, multiple marriages were not uncommon among the Cheyenne Indians during the nineteenth century. An examination of the 1880 census reveals that of 127 families, 16.5% were polygynous (from the perspective of the husbands) (Moorehead, 1991). Of the 799 persons who constituted these families, 212, or 26.5%, were members of polygynous families (Moorehead, 1991).

Several previously-existing communal societies in the U.S. embraced group marriage including, for example, the Oneida community. This community was founded by the Congregationalist minister John Humphrey Noyes in 1848 in Oneida, New York, following his hasty departure from the irate citizens of Putney, Vermont, who were displeased with his teachings and actions (Klephart and Zellner, 1998). The community adopted Noyes' teachings of "Mutual Criticism," "Male Continence," and "Complex Marriage," meaning that marriage and private property were abolished and the community included "all property of family living and associations." Mutual Criticism meant that all members of the community were subject to criticisms of either a committee or the whole community. These criticisms, which focused on an individual's "bad traits," were intended to assure conformity to community morality. The principle of Male Continence maintained that a male and female were to engage in sexual intercourse without the male ejaculating, in order to avoid unwanted pregnancy and the waste of sperm.

Complex Marriage dictated that every man and woman were married to all others of the opposite sex in the community. A male and female could cohabit only if they obtained each other's consent through a third party. However, exclusive attachments were prohibited as selfish and idolatrous. Noyes regularly criticized the practice of monogamy:

The human heart is capable of loving any number of times and any number of persons. This is the law of nature. There is no occasion to find fault with it. Variety is in the nature of things, as beautiful and as useful in love as in eating and drinking . . . . We need love as much as we need food and clothing, and God knows it; and if we trust Him for those things, why not for love? (Quoted in Parker, 1935: 182-183).

The *Handbook* of the community explained further the concept of sex within the community:

The liberty of monogamous marriage, as commonly understood, is the liberty of a man to sleep habitually with a woman, liberty to please himself alone in his dealings with her, liberty to expose her to childbearing without care or consultation.

The term Free Love, as understood by the Oneida Community, does not mean any such freedom of sexual proceedings. The theory of sexual interchange which governs all the general measures of the Community is that which in ordinary society governs the proceedings in courtship.

It is the theory that love after marriage should be what it is before marriage—a glowing attraction on both sides, and not the odious obligation of one party, and the sensual recklessness of the other (Quoted in Kephart and Zellner, 1998: 77).

The principle of "Ascending Fellowship" helped to guide the choice of sexual partner. This principle permitted older Central Members, deemed to be closer to God, to select younger virginal sexual partners to introduce them to the concept of Complex Marriage. Female Central Members were postmenopausal in order to prevent unwanted pregnancies. The selected virginal male or female was required to accept his or her selection, being of lower order (Hillebrand, n.d.).

The Oneida community was premised, in part, on religious belief. Community members believed that Christ's second coming had occurred in A.D. 70 and that they could bring in the millennium kingdom themselves. At its peak, the community had 306 members. The community was ultimately abandoned in 1881 due to internal community conflict arising in response to the policies imposed by Dr. Theodore Noyes, the founder's agnostic son, who assumed leadership from his father in 1876.

Several writers have noted that relative scarcity of African American men available for marital partnering to African American women (Chapman, 1986; Scott, 1976; Williams, 1990), due to high homicide rates, high rates of imprisonment, high rates of military service in response to the unavailability of adequate civilian employment, and the increasing rates of marriage between African American men and non-African American women (Williams, 1990). Polygyny, signifying here the establishment of "socio-sexual and even conjugal-type relationships" between multiple women and one male, has been proposed as a solution to this dilemma (Scott, 1976; cf. Chapman, 1986). At least one writer has argued against this approach, noting the preference of most women for unions between one man and one woman; the relative economic instability of many potentially available, marriageable African American men, thereby obviating their ability to provide for multiple households or persons; the health risks possibly associated with multiple partnering: and the existence of legal prohibitions against the recognition of multiple formalized, legal unions (Williams, 1990).

Finally, a proportion of the U.S. population today participates in various forms of multi-bonded relationships (Cloud, 1999; Strassberg, 2003), as evidenced by the number of websites, such as that for the Polyamory Society (http://www.polyamorysociety.org, last accessed December 8, 2004), and publications, such as *Loving More Magazine*, dedicated to multi-partnering. These relationships may vary in the level of commitment of each of the individuals to the relationship members, and the sexual or nonsexual nature of the interactions between each of the various individuals (Nearing, 1992; West, 1996).

Multi-bonding Across Cultures: Case Examples

As indicated, attitudes towards the bonding of multiple parties concurrently varies across cultures and societies and may range from encouragement of and support for formalized multi-party unions to the imposition of legal sanctions. Within this broad spectrum, societies may accept, tolerate, or decry less formal arrangements, such as sexual relationships outside of a primary, legally sanctioned relationship. This section examines the occurrence of multiple unions in three diverse settings and communities: Mormons in the United States and Bedouin-Arabs in Israel.

Multiple Marriage and the Church of the Latter Day Saints

The practice of multiple marriage was introduced into the Church of the Latter Day Saints (LDS) in the 1830s and 1840s, following the Church's relocation from the Midwest to the Great Basin. In 1852, Brigham Young announced that plural marriage would be the official doctrine of the Church (Batchelor, Watson, and Wilde, 2000). Both Mormons and non-Mormons of this time referred to the system of a man's marriage to more than one woman as "polygamy," "celestial marriage," "plural marriage," "plurality," and "the principle," (Hardy and Erickson, 2001), while Mormons also referred to plural marriage as "The Law of Abraham" and "patriarchal marriage" (Batchelor, Watson, and Wilde, 2000). Various arguments were presented to support the practice. Sexual activity for the purpose of reproduction was encouraged, while early death would befall those who engaged in too frequent sexual intercourse or intercourse with partners who could not conceive. Brigham Young subscribed to the then-prevalent notion that men possessed a greater sexual need and capacity than did women, so that multiple wives would serve both the men and women involved in the relationship and further a life in harmony (Hardy and Erickson, 2001).

Church doctrine has also been proffered to support the practice of polygamous marriage. The *Journal of Discourses (J.D.)*, a 26-volume collection of sermons and discourses delivered by LDS leaders during the period from 1853 through 1886, advises

God never introduced the Patriarchal order of marriage with a view to please man in his carnal desires, nor to punish females for anything which they had done; but He introduced it for the express purpose of raising up to His name a royal Priesthood, a peculiar people (Brigham Young, J.D. 3:264).

Now if any of you will deny the plurality of wives, and continue to do so, I promise that you will be damned; . . . (Brigham Young, J.D. 3: 266).

I want to prophesy that all men and women who oppose the revelation which God has given in relation to polygamy will find themselves in darkness, the spirit of God will withdraw from them the very moment of their opposition to that principle, until they will finally go down to hell and be damned, if they do not repent (Orson Pratt, J.D. 17: 224)

Estimates place the proportion of Mormon men who ever practiced polygamy as low as 3% and as high as 30% (Kephart and Zellner, 1998). Of those who did practice polygamy, it appears that the majority took only one additional wife. Those that did were most often in the upper economic strata.

Many Mormon women, as well as men, supported polygamy as an institution. It was believed that parents' thoughts could be passed on to their unborn child, and that women's emotions could be imprinted on their infants during gestation and nursing. Accordingly, some women believed that the emotional distress that they suffered in response to their husbands' imprisonment for polygamy would leave marks on their unborn children (Jensen, 1948).

It has been said that women who subscribe to plural marriage are convinced of 10 basic beliefs: (1) that plural marriage is a divine and holy law and is absolutely essential in order to receive the promised rewards; (2) that it is essential for her to live a plural marriage in this life; (3) that a monogamous marriage is insufficient for her to achieve the promised rewards; (4) that plural marriage is the only type of marriage that can continue beyond death; (5) that God has provided a way for her to practice plural marriage legitimately now; (6) that plural marriage is a holy principle; (7) that plural marriage is one of the laws that God designed to help her achieve her full potential, including her status as a goddess and her husband as a god; (8) that plural marriage is an eternal and essential component of the LDS religion, existing within a framework of personal covenants with God which bind individuals and families into a covenant people; (9) that she will receive huge rewards for living plural marriage; and (10) that she is entitled to divine, personal direction throughout her life (Anon., 2000: 71-72). Wives in polygamous marriages have identified numerous advantages of this marital arrangement as compared to monogamy, including the existence of multiple mothers to care for children, the establishment of close relationships with the other wives, the achievement of individual happiness and fulfillment of personal goals, and avoidance of marital problems resulting from a partner's adulterous affairs (Batchelor, Watson, and Wilde, 2000).

Various pieces of federal legislation were formulated to prohibit polygamy. Ultimately, LDS members adopted a Manifesto that advised church members to refrain from engaging in polygamy and Utah adopted a state constitution prohibiting polygamy in exchange for Utah's statehood. However, the Church hierarchy continued to encourage plural marriages, which prompted congressional hearings and a refusal by Congress in 1904 to allow the newly elected Utah Senator Reed Smoot, an LDS member, to take his seat in Congress (Batchelor, Watson, and Wilde, 2000). Ultimately, Church leadership promulgated the Second Manifesto, reaffirming that no polygamous marriages would be performed with the approval or consent of the Church.

Since that time, polygamous marriages that have occurred have been entered into outside of the authority of the Church and outside of the law. A number of these relationships have resulted in the prosecution of the adults involved, as well as trials relating to the fitness of the parents to retain custody of their children (*Sanderson v. Tryon*, 1987). Current Utah law prohibits polygamous or plural marriages (Utah Const.; Utah Code Ann., 2004), marriage of a child under the age of 16, in most cases (Utah Code Ann., 2004), and imposes criminal penalties on those who engage in bigamy (Utah Code Ann., 2004). However, various newspaper articles continue to document the occurrence of "marriages" involving one husband and multiple wives, despite the existing legal prohibitions and the fact that such marriages are legally void. In addition, these accounts have noted instances of abuse of multiple wives by Fundamentalist Mormons practicing polygamy, as well as the sexual abuse of female children, who were alleged to have been forced into early marriages.

The Bedouin-Arabs

The term "Bedouin," now used to refer to all Arabic-speaking nomadic tribes in the Middle East, was once reserved as a term of reference for those people who herded camels (Kay, 1978). Although the Bedouin Arabs of the Negev region are related to Bedouin communities in other countries, they comprise a distinct national, linguistic, political, and geographic group. The majority of the Bedouin living in the Negev region are Muslims, although there are some Christian Bedouins who live outside of this area. Of the approximately 100,000 Bedouins currently living in the Negev, approximately 40% live in villages and another 60% live semi-nomadically in rural areas (Al-Krenawi and Graham, 1997).

Bedouin society is founded on a tribal structure. These tribes are divided into units of various sizes based on kinship and patrilineal descent. The largest unit is that of a confederation or nation, which is comprised of various tribes grouped together; although each tribe has its own settlement, this association of the tribes provides a sense of belonging. A tribe consists of a union of families who wander together and work the land together under the rule of the tribal leader. In turn, the tribes may include smaller social groups, such as numbers of extended families, or *Hamula*. The *Hamula* encompass several generations in a patrilineal line that have a common ancestor. Marriages often involve unions between members of the *Hamula*.

Each *Hamula* has a representative, usually the eldest male, in the forum that makes the decisions in the tribe. Reports indicate that the man is usually the dominant figure in the tribe, is responsible for the family's relationships with others, and is the final authority in all matters related to his family (Al-Krenawi, 1996; Al-Krenawi, Maoz, and Riecher, 1994). The society is reported to be extremely hierarchical, with males dominant over females and older age over younger age. Family members are tied together culturally, socially, economically, and emotionally and are expected to assist each other (Al-Krenawi and Graham, 1996).

Because traditional Bedouin-Arab society was organized as warrior tribes, the roles of males and females were strictly delineated. As a consequence, sons have higher status and more value than daughters. Women are referred to as *Aorah*, which means literally, "disabled." (Al-Krenawi, 1998). A woman's status in this society is dependent upon her marital status and her production of children, especially sons. Polygamy remains common and more than four wives have been known to be acquired, despite the numerical limitation imposed by the Koran (Al-Krenawi, 1996). Marriages are often arranged by a girl's family while she is still in her teens, frequently without her consultation. Women are expected to remain in the home and to forego higher education, while men are expected to be the breadwinners. Women are deemed to be the property of the man of the family; their good behavior upholds his honor (Al-Krenawi, 1998).

Divorce often results in serious emotional and economic consequences. The husband is entitled to the custody of the children in the event of divorce, regardless of the children's ages (Al-Krenawi, 1996; Mass and Al-Krenawi, 1994). A divorced woman may have no means of support other than assistance from other family members or court-ordered support payments from her ex-husband (Al-Krenawi, 1998). Once divorced, she will be able to remarry only as a second, third, or fourth wife or as the wife of an older man (Al-Krenawi, 1996).

Multi-bonding and Health

Fertility

The effect of male coupling with multiple women on fertility remains unsettled (Dodoo, 1998). A number of researchers have asserted that polygynous relationships do not result in a reduction in fertility (Lorimer, 1954; Nag, 1962), while others claim to have observed a reduction (Henin, 1968; Morgan, 1971; Ukaegbu,

1977; Van de Walle, 1968). The apparent observed reduction in fertility has been explained by the existence of a wide age disparity between male and his younger wives, such that the male's ability to procreate has declined significantly and continues to decrease, resulting in a reduction in the fertility of successive wives (Ukaegbu, 1977).

Women and Health

Scholars have variously perceived women in polygynous unions as incapable of relating to each other except through competition (Pogrebin, 1987) or as establishing cooperation and friendship in an effort to empower themselves against male control and domination (Smith-Rosenberg, 1975). However, studies of polygyny across cultures suggest that women's attitudes towards polygyny may vary within and across societies (Adams and Mburugu, 1994; Dorjahn, 1988; Kilbride, 1994; Potash, 1989; White and Burton, 1988) and that their experiences and perspectives can only be understood within a particular sociocultural and personal context (Madhavan, 2002).

Various researchers have found in their studies of African societies that polygyny may be advantageous for women in some societies because polygynous husbands tend to be wealthier, the pool of laborers available for work as a function of the larger domestic unit reduces the need for wage laborers, and co-wives may provide assistance with labor and in economic affairs (Adams and Mburugu, 1994; Dorjahn, 1988). Ware's (1979) study of Yoruba women's attitudes towards polygyny found that approximately 60% favored a polygynous arrangement because it would provide both a social opportunity to gossip and play, as well as assistance with the domestic labor. Polygynous unions may also provide an alternative to divorce in those societies in which marriage is determinative of women's status and/or divorce results in stigmatization or ostracism (Al-Krenawi, Graham, and Slonim-Nevo, 2002).

Kinship, norms about friendship, and closer age of the co-wives may be critical factors in the formation of a friendship or collaborative relationship between various co-wives (Madhavan, 2002). For instance, older women may expect newer, younger wives to adapt to the status quo. Too, societal expectations regarding the nature of co-wife relationships may play an important role. As an example, the Bamanan community of Mali expects that existing wives will accept their husband's acquisition of additional wives, while the Fulbe community of Mali anticipates jealousy between co-wives and competition to keep the man (Madhavan, 2002).

Studies of polygynous relationships in Africa have also, however, documented significant difficulties. Wives may not welcome the entry of new co-wives into the relationship, fearing that their inclusion will result in a reduction in the availability of material resources for themselves and their children, a diminution in their husband's emotional availability to themselves and their children, and/or a reduction in their husband's sexual availability (Adams and Mburugu, 1994; Ware, 1979, Wittrup, 1990). Such fears or perceptions may give rise to envy and jealousy between co-wives (Eichenbaum and Orbach, 1988; Fainzang and Journet, 1988; Potash, 1995). Although some reports and accounts indicate that wife order may be an important factor in women's satisfaction in their relationship (Chaleby, 1985), a study of polygamous marriages in Cameron found that wife order had a negligible effect on either life or marital satisfaction among the women (Gwanfogne, Furrow, Schumm, and Smith, 1997).

Even where there exists significant social support for the institution of polygyny, women may disfavor it, feeling that it is in their best interest and the best interests of their children to oppose their husband's inclination to acquire an additional wife (Meekers and Franklin, 1995). Despite such opposition, however, women may ultimately feel powerless to prevent its occurrence (Meekers and Franklin, 1995). Women may also resign themselves to the possibility that their husbands will take additional wives to avoid a more distasteful alternative: that their husbands will be legally monogamous but will engage in a series of affairs. An interview study with 250 wives in Nigeria found that three-quarters of the wives preferred that their husbands take an additional wife rather than a mistress, noting that men spend less money on their wives than their mistresses and that the position of an additional wife was more defined and controllable than that of a mistress (Ware, 1979).

Although the potential exists for women in a polygynous union to be at an economic disadvantage due to the sharing of available resources, such an adverse result may not occur. For instance, Hames (1996) found in his study of the Yanomamö Indians of Venezuela that these potential economic costs of polygyny are avoided by the provision of subsidies to polygynous households by other households in the village, as a function of the high status held by the husbands in such unions.

A study of women in an inpatient psychiatric facility in Kuwait found that almost one-quarter of the patients were members of polygamous marriages, although slightly more than one-tenth of married women in the general population were members of such marriages (Chaleby, 1985). The ratio of senior to junior wives in the psychiatric population was 2 to 1; the ratio increased to 3 to 1 when cases of mental illness arising before the second marriage were excluded from the analysis. Depression was more frequently diagnosed among polygamous than monogamous wives and among senior as compared with junior wives. Multiple explanations may have existed for these findings, however, including an increased incidence of mental illness among polygamous wives, a desire on the part of the husbands to discard the senior wives, and/or the wives' use of hospitalization as a means of escaping from restrictions and responsibilities imposed by the family structure. The increased frequency of depression among senior wives may have been attributable to older age depression associated with hormonal changes and/or feelings of loss engendered by the husbands' acquisition of additional wives (Chaleby, 1985).

A similar study of psychiatric outpatients found that 25.4% were in polygamous marriages, compared to an estimated 11.5% of all married women based upon data from the 1975 Kuwaiti census and estimates from marriage court statistics (Chaleby, 1987). Lower levels of education and unemployment were associated with being in a polygamous marriage. Polygamous wives were more likely than those in monogamous marriages to attribute their psychiatric disorders to their marital status. Although not raised as a possibility by the researchers, one must consider whether the polygamous marriages and lack of education and employment were effects of the mental illness. It is possible, for instance, that the mental illness precluded the women from advancing educationally and securing and retaining employment. Too, the mental illness may have limited the extent to which the women could assume responsibility for the management of a household and the care of its members.

Several studies have examined the frequency of polygamy among mentally ill patients in Nigeria, where polygamy has been found to be relatively common (Makanjuola, 1987). Of 318 patients in Ilesha, it was found that 81% had been born into polygamous homes (Makanjuola, 1985). An earlier study of psychiatric disorders among the Yoruba found that mental disorder occurred more frequently among co-wives in the city, but not in the village (Leighton, Lambo, Hughes, Leighton, Murphy, and Macklin, 1963).

Not surprisingly, monogamous wives may experience greater pressure to satisfy their husbands' sexual demands than do polygamous wives. Monogamous wives may be more "yielding" due to fears that if they fail or refuse to satisfy their husbands, their husbands will take another wife or engage in extramarital affairs (Ware, 1979).

Better educated and urban women have been found to be less likely to favor polygyny (Ferraro, 1991, Klomegah, 1997; Okonjo, 1992; Ware, 1979; Wittrup, 1990). Not surprisingly, then, the proportion of marriages in Africa that are polygynous has declined due to an increase in women's education, urbanization, and changes in women's status (Madhavan, 2002). However, informal polygyny, whereby a man maintains one or more extramarital relationships, has become increasingly common (Potash, 1995).

One must necessarily inquire about the relevance of these findings in African societies to relationship dynamics in the United States, where multiple legal marriage remains illegal. An interview study with 17 American Muslim women of diverse backgrounds reported similar difficulties (Hassouneh-Phillips, 2000). The women, many of whom were first wives, became unwilling participants in polygamous relationships. The women reported unequal distributions of time, financial support, and affection among wives. Although a number of the marriages involved physical abuse by the husbands, co-wives did not attempt to intervene to assist each other in such circumstances and, in some instances, were co-perpetrators of the abuse.

It is possible that the illegal status of polygamous relationships in the United States may also play a role in the effect of the relationship structure on women's mental health. One woman who left a fundamentalist Mormon community that practiced polygamy wrote:

In the polygamous culture, personal identity is hard to come by. Social boundaries around the religious group keep out the larger world, but inside the group, personal boundaries are discouraged and readily breached. The secrecy imposed by an illegal lifestyle further undermines individual development, increasing the likelihood of abuse and exploitation. Focus on the self is actively discouraged . . . (Solomon, 2003: 13).

Men's Health

Little attention has focused specifically on the effect of multiple-bonded partnerships on the health of the males involved in these partnerships. An early study of Yoruba men found that married men with more than one wife were less likely to be mentally ill than those who had only one wife (Leighton, Lambo, Hughes, Leighton, Murphy, and Macklin, 1963). The researchers hypothesized that having only one wife was an effect, rather than a cause, of mental illness and that a degree of premorbid instability made these men less able to attract potential spouses.

Child Development

Relatively few studies of child development in the context of multi-bonding, regardless of its form, are available. Despite extensive theorizing about the negative impact of a polygamous family structure on the behavioral, emotional, and academic adjustment of children (Elbedour, Onwuegbuzie, Caridine, and Abu-Saad, 2002), we actually have very little empirical data related to these questions.

Researchers have hypothesized that polygyny represents a male reproductive strategy that permits men to maximize the number of children, while minimizing their investment in each child (White, 1988). As a result, various investigations have been conducted in an attempt to discern differences in child development as a function of the marital structure of the family.

A number of recent studies have centered on a comparison of polygamous and monogamous Bedouin-Arab families in Israel (Al-Krenawi, Graham, and Al-Krenawi, 1997; Al-Krenawi, Graham, and Slonim-Nevo, 2002; Al-Krenawi and Lightman, 2000; Elbedour, Bart, and Hektner, 2000, 2003). Comparisons of the children's development by family structure have yielded conflicting findings. A study of adolescents from polygamous and monogamous Bedouin-Arab families in the Negev area of Israel found no significant differences in adolescent intelligence measures (Elbedour, Bart, and Hektner, 2003) or in scholastic achievement (Elbedour, Bart, and Hektner, 2000). However, other researchers have reported comparatively lower academic achievement levels among children from polygamous families (Al-Krenawi, Graham, and Al-Krenawi, 1997; Al-Krenawi, Graham, and Slonim-Nevo, 2002; Al-Krenawi and Lightman, 2000; Cherian, 1989). At least one research group attributed the reduced academic achievement in polygamous households to a reduced level of parental interest in their children, regardless of the form of marriage (Cherian, 1993).

Adolescent levels of self-esteem have been found to be diminished (Al-Krenawi, Graham, and Slonim-Nevo, 2002; Owuamanam, 1984), levels of depression have been found to be higher (Al-Krenawi, Graham, and Slonim-Nevo, 2002), and behavioral difficulties in school more frequent (Minde, 1975) in children of polygynous unions as compared to those of monogamous unions. Investigators have hypothesized that the difficulties experienced by adolescents of polygynous unions with respect to self-esteem and self-identity may be related both to the tensions between their mothers, other co-wives, and their father and to a perceived or real lack of attention from their fathers (Al-Krenawi, Graham, and Slonim-Nevo, 2002; Owuamanam, 1984; Oyefoso and Adegoke, 1992). An investigation of the psychological adjustment of 116 Yoruba adolescents found that among males, but not among females, psychological adjustment as measured by the Psychological Adjustment Scale was significantly worse for those in polygynous households as compared with those in monogamous families (Oyefoso and Adegoke, 1992).

A case study of two situations involving informal polygamy focused on a child's behavioral problems. The therapists involved ultimately concluded that the difficulties experienced by the "problem child" in each family were not attributable to the family structure, but instead resulted from factors such as parental inconsistencies and a lack of contact between the one family, consisting of the man and his legal wife, and the second family, consisting of the same man and the family resulting from his informal polygamous union (Rivett and Street, 1993).

Implications for Research and Practice

This chapter examined various forms of multi-bonding, with a particular focus on formalized polygyny. This brief review underscores our relative lack of knowledge with respect to many basic questions. These include: Why does there appear, at least in some instances, to be a higher proportion of wives in polygamous, as opposed to monogamous, relationships among mentally ill patients? Why does increased education appear to decrease women's willingness to enter into polygamous unions? What are the effects of multi-bonding on men's physical and mental health? What environmental factors impact the success or failure of individuals' effort to engage in multi-bonding? How do these same environmental factors affect the adjustment of children raised in multi-bonded families?

Multi-bonding raises critical issues in the clinical context, as well. Many practitioners might assume that a "married" man or woman, at least in the United States, is "married" to only one individual. In fact, various partnering configurations may potentially exist. In most cases, it is likely that a patient or client would not be willing to disclose the fact of such alternative arrangements to a clinician, unless there had developed a basis for trust and mutual respect. It is critical, then, that practitioners, regardless of their discipline, attempt to understand the social, cultural, and religious context in which their patient or client operates and engage the patient or client in discussion of his or her situation in that context. This clearly becomes increasingly difficult as the time available for patient examinations and client appointments continues to be diminished due to the constraints imposed by managed care health care systems.

References

Adams, B., Mburugu, E. (1994). Kikuyu bridewealth and polygyny today. *Journal of Comparative Family Studies* 25(2): 159-166.

Al-Krenawi, A. (1998). Family therapy with a multiparental/multi-spousal family. *Family Process* 37: 65-81.

Al-Krenawi, A. (1996). Group work with Bedouin widows of the Negev in a medical clinic. *Affilia: Journal of Women and Social Work* 11: 303-318.

Al-Krenawi, A., Graham, R.J. (1996). Social work among the Bedouin of the Negev, Israel. *International Social Work* 39: 177-188.

Al-Krenawi, A., Graham, R.J. (1997). Spirit possession and exorcism: The integration of modern and traditional mental health care systems in the treatment of a Bedouin patient. *Clinical Social Work Journal* 25: 211-222.

Al-Krenawi, A., Graham, J.R., Al-Krenawi, S. (1997). Social work practice with polygamous families. *Child and Adolescent Social Work Journal* 14(6): 445-458.

Al-Krenawi, A., Graham, J.R., Slonim-Nevo, V. (2002). Mental health aspects of Arab-Israeli adolescents from polygamous versus monogamous families. *Journal of Social Psychology* 142(4): 446-460.

Al-Krenawi, A., Lightman, E.S. (2000). Learning achievement, social adjustment, and family conflict among Bedouin-Arab children from polygamous and monogamous families. *Journal of Social Psychology* 140(3): 345-355.

Al-Krewnawi, A., Maoz, B., Riecher, B. (1994). Familial and cultural issues in the brief strategic treatment of Israeli Bedouin. Family Systems Medicine 12: 415-425.

Altman, I., Ginat, J. (1996). *Polygamous Families in Contemporary Society*. Cambridge, U.K.: Cambridge University Press.

Anon. (2004). Group marriage. Wikipedia. Available at http://en.wikipedia.org/wiki/Group_marriage. Last accessed August 17, 2004.

Anon. (2000). Why do women choose plural marriage?: A guest essay by an anonymous plural wife. In M. Batchelor, M. Watson, A. Wilde (Eds.). *Voices in Harmony: Contemporary Women Celebrate Plural Marriage* (pp. 70-74). Salt Lake City, Utah: Principle Voices.

Batchelor, M., Watson, M., Wilde, A. (Eds.). (2000). *Voices in Harmony: Contemporary Women Celebrate Plural Marriage.* Salt Lake City, Utah: Principle Voices.

Chaleby, K. (1985). Women of polygamous marriages in an inpatient psychiatric services in Kuwait. *Journal of Nervous and Mental Disease* 173(1): 56-58.

Chaleby, K. (1987). Women of polygamous marriages in outpatient psychiatric services in Kuwait. *International Journal of Family Psychiatry* 8(1): 25-34.

Chapman, A. (1986). *Man Sharing, Dilemma or Choice: A Radical New Way of Relating to the Men in Your Life.* New York: William Morrow.

Cherian, V.I. (1989). Academic achievement of children from monogamous and polygynous families. *Journal of Social Psychology* 130(1): 117-119.

Cherian, V.I. (1993). The relationship between parental interest and academic achievement of Xhosa children from monogamous and polygynous families. *Journal of Social Psychology* 133(5): 733-736.

Cloud, J. (1999). Henry & Mary & Janet & . . . . *Time Magazine*, Nov. 15, 154(20).

Dodoo, F.N.A. (1998). Marriage type and reproductive decisions: A comparative study in Sub-Saharan Africa. *Journal of Marriage and the Family* 60: 232-242.

Dorjahn, V.R. (1988). Changes in Temne polygyny. *Ethnology* 27: 367-390.

Dorjahn, V.R. (1959). The factor of polygyny in African demography. In W.R. Bascom, M.J. Herskovits (Eds.). *Continuity and Change in African Cultures* (pp. 87-112). Chicago: University of Chicago Press.

Eichenbaum, L., Orbach, S. (1988). *Between Women: Love, Envy, and Competition in Women's Friendships.* New York: Viking Press.

El Azayem G.A., Hedayat-Diba, Z. (1994). The psychological aspects of Islam: Basic principles of Islam and their psychological corollary. *The International Journal for the Psychology of Religion* 4(1): 41-50.

Elbedour, S., Bart, W.M., Hektner, J.M. (2003). Intelligence and family marital structure: The case of adolescents from monogamous and polygamous families among Bedouin Arabs in Israel. *Journal of Social Psychology* 143(1): 95-110.

Elbedour, S., Bart, W.M., Hektner, J.M. (2000). Scholastic achievement and family marital structure: Bedouin-Arab adolescents from monogamous and polygamous families in Israel. *Journal of Social Psychology* 140(4): 503-514.

Elbedour, S., Onwuegbuzie, A.J., Caridine, C., Abu-Saad, H. (2002). The effect of polygamous marital structure on behavioral, emotional, and academic adjustment in children: A comprehensive review of the literature. *Clinical Child and Family Psychology Review* 5(4): 255-271.

Fainzang, S., Journet, O. (1988). La Femme de Mon Mari. Paris. Cited in S. Madhavan. Best of friends and worst of enemies: Competition and collaboration in polygyny. *Ethnology* 41(1): 69-84.

Ferraro, G.P. (1991). Marriage and conjugal roles in Swaziland: Persistence and change. *International Journal of Sociology of the Family* 21(2): 89-128.

Grønstøol, G.B., Byrkjedal, I., Fiksen, Ø. (2003). Predicting polygynous settlement while incorporating varying female competitive strength. *Behavioral Ecology* 14(2): 257-267.

Gwanfoghe, P.N., Furrow, J.L., Schumm, W.R., Smith, M. (1997). Polygamy and marital life satisfaction: An exploratory study from rural Cameroon. *Journal of Comparative Family Studies* 28(1): 55-71.

Hames, R. (1996). Costs and benefits of monogamy and polygyny for Yanomamö women. *Ethology and Sociobiology* 17: 181-199.

Haqqi, S.A.H. (1974). Polygamy among Indian Muslims: A case study. *Indian Journal of Politics* 8: 143-152.

Hardy, R.C., Erickson, D. (2001). "Regeneration—Now and evermore": Mormon polygamy and the physical rehabilitation of mankind. *Journal of the History of Sexuality* 10(1): 40-61.

Hassouneh-Phillips, D. (2001). Polygamy and wife-abuse: A qualitative study of Muslim women in America. *Health Care for Women International* 22: 735-748.

Henin, R.A. (1968). Fertility differentials in the Sudan. *Population Studies* 12: 147-161.

Hillebrand, R. (n.d.). The Oneida community. New York History Net. Available at http://www.nyhistory.com/central/oneida,htm. Last accessed August 16, 2004.

Hillman, E. (1975). *Polygyny Reconsidered.* New York: Orbis Books.

Jensen J.B. (1948). *Little God Pieces: The Story of My Mormon Mother's Life.* Salt Lake City, Utah.

Kephart, W.M., Zellner, W.W. (1998). *Extraordinary Groups: An Examination of Unconventional Lifestyles.* New York: St. Martin's Press.

Kilbride, P. (1994). *Plural Marriage for Our Times: A Reinvented Option.* Westport, Connecticut: Greenwood Publishing Group.

Klomegah, R. (1997). Socio-economic characteristics of Ghanaian women in polygamous marriages. *Journal of Comparative Family Studies* 28: 73-89.

Lauras-Lecoh, T. (1990). Family trends and demographic transition in Africa. *International Social Science Journal* 42(4): 475-492.

Lee, G.R. (1979). Marital structure and economic systems. *Journal of Marriage and the Family* 41: 701-713.

Leighton, A.H., Lambo, T.A., Hughes, C.C., Leighton, D.C., Murphy, J.M., Macklin, H.B. (1963). *Psychiatric Disorder among the Yoruba.* New York: Cornell University Press.

Lesthaeghe, R., Kaufmann, G., Meekers, D. (1987). Marriage patterns and change in Sub-Saharan Africa. In J.A. Ebigbola, E. Van de Walle (Eds.). The Cultural Roots of African Fertility Regimes. University of Ile-Ife and University of Pennsylvania. Cited in T. Lauras-Lecoh. (1990). Family trends and demographic transition in Africa. *International Social Science Journal* 42(4): 475-492.

Lorimer, F. (Ed.). (1954). *Culture and Human Fertility.* Paris: UNESCO.

Madhavan, S. (2002). Best of friends and worst of enemies: Competition and collaboration in polygyny. *Ethnology* 41(1): 69-84.

Makanjuola, R.O.A. (1985). Clinical and sociocultural parameters in Nigerian psychiatric patients: A prospective study. *Acta Psychiatrica Scandinavia* 72: 512-521.

Makanjuola, R.O.A. (1987). The Nigerian psychiatric patient and his family. *International Journal of Family Psychiatry* 8(4): 363-373.

Mass, M., Al-Krenawi, A. (1994). When a man encounters a woman, Satan is also present: Clinical relationships in Bedouin society. *American Journal of Orthopsychiatry* 64: 357-367.

Meekers, D., Franklin, N. (1995). Women's perceptions of polygyny among the Kaguru of Tanzania. *Ethnology* 34(4): 315-329.

Minde, K.K. (1975). Psychological problems in Ugandan school children: A controlled evaluation. *Journal of Child Psychology and Psychiatry* 16: 49-59.

Misovich, S.J., Fisher, J.D., Fisher, W.A. (1997). Close relationships and elevated risk behavior: Evidence and possibly underlying psychological processes. *Review of General Psychology* 1(1): 72-107.

Momeni, D.A. (1975). Polygyny in Iran. *Journal of Marriage and the Family* 37(2): 453-456.

Moorehead, J. H. (1991). The developmental cycle of Cheyenne polygyny. *American Indian Quarterly* 15(3): 311-328.

Munson, M., Stelboum J. Introduction. In M. Munson, J.P. Stelboum (Eds.). *The Lesbian Polyamory Reader: Open Relationships, Non-Monogamy, and Casual Sex* (pp. 1-7). New York: Haworth Press, Inc., 1999.

Murdock, G.P. (1949). *Social Structure*. New York: Macmillan.

Nag, M. (1962). *Factors Affecting Fertility in Non-Industrial Societies: A Cross-Cultural Study*. New Haven: Yale University Publications in Anthropology.

Nearing, R. (1992). *Loving More: The Polyfidelity Primer*. Hawaii: PEP Publications.

Okonjo, K. (1992). Aspects of continuity and change in mate-selection among the Igbo west of the Niger River. *Journal of Comparative Family Studies* 23(3): 339-360.

Oyefoso, A.O., Adegoke, A.R. (1992). Psychological adjustment of Yoruba adolescents as influenced by family type: A research note. *Journal of Child Psychology and Psychiatry* 33(4): 785-788.

Owuamanam, D.O. (1984). Adolescents' perception of polygamous family and its relationship to self-concept. *International Journal of Psychology* 19: 593-598.

Parker, R. (1935). *Yankee Saint: John Humphrey Noyes and the Oneida Community*. New York: Putnam.

Pitshandege, N. (1978). De la polygamie et fécondité dans la sociéteé zaîroise: L'example des Yaka de la zone de Popokabaka. Working Paper

No. 57, Département de Démographie, Université Catholique de Louvain. Cited in C.E. Welch III & P.C. Glick (1981). The incidence of polygamy in contemporary Africa: A research note. *Journal of Marriage and the Family* 43(1):191-193.

Potash, B. (1989). Gender relations in Sub-Saharan Africa. In S. Morgan (Ed.). *Gender and Anthropology: Critical Reviews for Teaching and Research* (pp. 189-227). Washington, D.C.: American Anthropological Association.

Potash, B. (1995). Women in the changing African family. M.J. Hay, S. Stichter (Eds.). *African Women: South of the Sahara* (pp. 69-92). Essex, U.K.: Addison-Wesley.

Ptak, S.E., Lachmann, L. (2003). On the evolution of polygyny: A theoretical examination of the polygyny threshold model. *Behavioral Ecology* 14(2): 201-211.

Rivett, M., Street, E. (1993). 'Informal polygamy': A suitable case for treatment? *Journal of Family Therapy* 15: 71-79.

Sanderson v. Tryon, 739 P.2d 623 (S. Ct. 1987).

Scott, J.W. (1976). Polygamy: A futuristic family arrangement for African-American. *Black Books Bulletin* 4(2): 13-19.

Smith-Rosenberg, C. (1975). The female world of love and ritual: Relations between women in nineteenth century America. *Sign* 1: 1-29.

Solomon, D.A. (2003). *Predators, Prey, and Other Kinfolk: Growing Up in Polygamy.* New York: W.W. Norton & Company.

Strassberg, M.I. (2003). The challenge of post-modern polygamy: Considering polyamory. *Capital University Law Review* 31: 439-563.

Tabutin, D. (1974). La polygamie en Algérie. *Population* 29: 313-326.

Uchendu, V.C. (1965). Concubinage among the Ngwa Igbo of Southern Nigeria. *Journal of the International African Institute* 35: 187-197.

Ukaegbu, A.O. (1977). Fertility of women of polygynous unions in rural Eastern Nigeria. *Journal of Marriage and the Family* 39(2): 397-404.

Utah Code Ann. §§ 30-1-2, 76-7-101 (2004).

Utah Const. Art. III and Ordinance (2004).

Van de Walle, E. (1968). Marriage in African censuses and inquiries. In W. Brass, A.J. Coale, P. Demeny, D.F. Heisel, F. Lorimer, A.

Romaniuk, & E. Van de Walle (Eds.). *The Demography of Tropical Africa* (pp. 183-238). New Jersey: Princeton University Press.

Ware, H. (1979). Polygyny: Women's views in a transitional society, Nigeria 1975. *Journal of Marriage and the Family* 41(2): 185-195.

Welch III, C.E., Glick, P.C. (1981). The incidence of polygamy in contemporary Africa: A research note. *Journal of Marriage and the Family* 43(1):191-193.

West, C. (1996). *Lesbian Polyfidelity*. San Francisco: Booklegger Publications.

White, D.R., Burton, M.L. (1988). Causes of polygyny: Ecology, economy, kinship, and warfare. *American Anthropologist* 90(4): 871-887.

Williams, M.W. (1990). Polygamy and the declining male to female ratio in black communities: A social inquiry. *Black Families* (Jan.): 171-193.

Wittrup, I. (1990). Me and my husband's wife: An analysis of polygyny among Mandinka in the Gambia. *Folk* 32: 117-142.

CHAPTER 3

Child "Partnering": Incest, Pedophilia, and Child Marriage

Incest

Defining What We Mean

An incest taboo appears to exist within all societies (Héritier, 1999; Meiselman, 1988). However, how that taboo is operationalized varies across societies. And, just as the language that we use to describe partnering relationships fails to encompass the many nuances, dimensions, and varieties of partnering relationships, so too does the language we use to describe the occurrence of sexual relations between children and adults fail to encompass the multiplicity of circumstances and dimensions that may exist in such interactions. Does child sexual abuse, for instance, become incest only due to the blood or legal ties that exist between the parties, or is something else required?

Consider, for instance, variations across legal definitions of incest. The Criminal Code of Canada refers to incest only in conjunction with sexual intercourse between blood relatives of the first and second degree, although adopted children are also included (Greenspan and Rosenberg, 2000). Utah's statutory definition of incest permits intercourse between those related in the second degree and prohibits sexual relationships between stepparent and stepchild while the marriage creating the relationships exists (Utah Code Annotated, 2004). Neither of these legal provisions encompasses marriage; one could presumably marry an individual with one of the stated relationships and not commit incest unless sexual intercourse actually occurs. In contrast, Alabama's prohibition against incest does not refer to relations between cousins of any degree; first cousins are free to marry or to have sexual intercourse as apparently are aunts, uncles, nephews, and nieces by marriage (Code of Alabama, 2004). However, the relations contained in the statutory definition of incest—ancestors or descendants by blood or adoption, brothers and sisters of the whole or half-blood or by adoption, stepchildren or stepparents during the existence of the marriage creating the relationship, and aunts, uncles, nephews and nieces of the whole or half-blood—commit incest not only by engaging in sexual intercourse but also by entering into marriage alone, even absent sexual intercourse (Code of Alabama, 2004). California, like Alabama, permits marriage and sexual relations between cousins of the first degree (California Family Code, 2004).

Ambiguity is further compounded by variations in the use of the term "incest" in the context of research. As an example, Sgroi (1982) has defined "incestuous child sexual abuse" as "any form of sexual activity between a child and a parent, stepparent, sibling, extended family member or surrogate parent figure." Extended family members are said to include grandparents, uncles, and aunts, while surrogate figures include common-law spouses or foster parents (Neal, 1991). According to Neal (1991), the presence or absence of a blood relationship is of less significance than the psychological meaning of the relationship. This presumes, however, that all parties to the sexual activity attribute the same psychological meaning to their relationship.

Yet another research group has defined incest as "any kind of sexual exploitative contact that occurs between relatives" (Rudd and Herzberger, 1999). Unlike Sgroi's definition, this definition encompasses all relatives, regardless of the nature of the relationship tie (blood or legal), degree of relation, or the age difference between the parties. Additionally, this second definition includes exploitation as a requisite element, thereby limiting the context in which sexual activity between the related individuals can be said to be incest. Accordingly, one must wonder whether, for instance, brother-sister sexual activity would constitute incest within the scope of this definition where the intent was simply to mimic behavior that the siblings had seen enacted by others or where the goal of the interaction between siblings was mutual pleasure or comfort. This definition can be contrasted with that used by Russell (1983) in a study of the experiences of San Francisco women: sexual contact, whether desired or not, with a relative at least 5 years older or unwanted sexual contact with any other relative. This definition omits from its scope behaviors such as exhibitionism and voyeurism, as well as desired sexual acts between related individuals who are within 5 years of age of each other. Still other definitions of incest that have been used in a research context limit the term's comprehensiveness by the age of the victim and/or the nature of the relationship between the persons involved. (See Table 1).

Conceptualizations of incest appear to intersect with those of child sexual abuse. The American Medical Association (1985: 798) has referred to the sexual abuse of children as the "exploitation of a child for gratification or profit of an adult," mirroring the definition of incest utilized by Rudd and Herzberger (1999) in referring to sexual activity between related persons. Alternative formulations appear to distinguish incest and child sexual abuse based upon the specific behaviors between the parties. Utah's incest law, for instance, has been interpreted to require actual contact of the sexual organs and penetration (Utah Code Annotated, 2004; *State v. Warner*, 1932). Similarly, some researchers omit specific behaviors from their definitions of incest; one research group did not consider covert sexual stimulation, such as fondling, French kissing, and explicit sexual discussions initiated by a father with an adolescent

Table 1. Sample of Definitions of Incest Used in Research Studies

Study	Definition of Incest
Caldirola et al., 1983	Does not include covert sexual stimulation, such as fondling, French kissing, explicit sexual discussions initiated by the parent
Ellenson, 1986	Any sexual contact between the perpetrator and the victim in which the perpetrator violated a position of trust or authority, with the first occurrence of the sexual contact taking place before the victim was 18 years of age
Finkelhor, 1979	Includes exhibition, fondling, petting, masturbation, oral-genital contact, or intercourse between family members
Laviola, 1992	Any sexual behavior that occurs between two family members, regardless of age differential, who are related by blood, marriage, or living arrangement
Owens, 1984	Includes intercourse, fondling, caressing, oral-genital relations, and mutual masturbation with biological fathers, stepfathers, mothers, siblings, uncles; the degree of relation with uncles unspecified
Rudd and Herzberger, 1999	Any kind of sexual exploitative contact that occurs between relatives
Russell, 1983	Sexual contact, whether desired or not, with a relative at least 5 years older than victim or unwanted sexual contact with any other relative
Sgroi, 1982	Incestuous child sexual abuse: Any form of sexual activity between a child and a parent, stepparent, sibling, extended family member or surrogate parent figure

Table 1. (*Continued*)

Study	Definition of Incest
Westerlund, 1992	Sexual activity between the child and a family member during childhood and/or adolescence. Sexual activity includes kissing, fondling, manipulation of the male and/or female genitalia, oral-genital contact, simulated intercourse, vaginal intercourse, anal intercourse, genital exhibition, masturbation by the adult in the presence of the child/adolescent, and peeping.

daughter to constitute incest (Caldirola, Gemperle, Guzinski, Gross, and Doerr, 1983).

Such behaviors, however, could potentially constitute sexual abuse of a child. Burton and Myers (1992) included the following acts in their definition of child sexual abuse: demanding or requesting nudity, disrobing, exposing genitals, observing a child dressing or bathing, kissing, and digitally or penilely penetrating the rectum or vagina. Sgroi (1982), however, merges the use of the two terms and their underlying concepts in referring to incestuous child abuse, which includes any form of sexual activity between specified relations. And if, as Neal (1991) postulates, the psychological significance of the relationship is really determinative of whether the behavior constitutes incest, then even sexual overtures to a child by a "friend of the family" could be classifiable as not only child sexual abuse, but also as incest.

Unfortunately, researchers who have examined or reviewed the etiology of adult-child sexual encounters and their consequences have all too often failed to distinguish between acts committed by relatives by blood, law, or surrogacy and those committed by non-related individuals (e.g., Arnow et al., 1999; Logan, Walker, Cole, and Leukefeld, 2002; Schetky, 1990). Others who have focused on incest have failed to specify the behaviors that are encompassed by their use of the term (e.g., Rice and Harris, 2002). As a result, we cannot know whether there are critical differences between the sequelae of sexual encounters with a child that are committed by a "related" individual and those committed by an individual without such an association. The existence of such differences may demand the formulation of distinct interventions, treatments, and preventive strategies. What is clear, however, is that, depending upon the definitions that are used, incest generally will be considered to be child sexual abuse, but not all sexual abuse of a child will be considered incest, due to either the nonexistence of a requisite relationship, the specific type of act that has occurred, and/or the absence of a requisite element, such as the intent to exploit. Ultimately, it may be only a minute proportion of all sexual acts engaged in with a child that can be said to constitute incest, as illustrated by the diagram below.

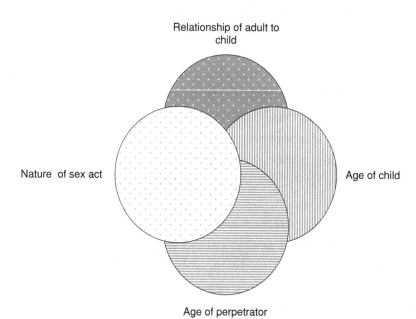

Figure 2. Relationship of Factors Utilized to Define Incest

Interactions occurring at the juncture of incest and child sexual abuse necessarily raise questions regarding the characteristics of the adult who engages in this behavior with children. Are adults who commit incestuous sexual acts similar to adults who engage in sexual activities with nonrelated children? Are they pedophiles? Research indicates that adults who engage in incestuous interactions show relatively less sexual interest in children than do those engaging in nonincestuous sexual relations with children (Seto, Lalumière, and Kuban, 1999). Additionally, biological fathers who have offended against their children have been found to be less sexually interested in children than men who offended against extended family members and have been found not to differ from stepfathers (Seto, Lalumière, and Kuban, 1999).

Incidence and Prevalence of Incest

Varying reports indicate that anywhere from 17% to 46% of children who are raped are raped by family members (Langan and Harlow, 1994; The National Treatment Center for Victims of Crimes and Crime Victims Research and Treatment Center, 1992). Herman's (1981) review of the literature indicated that between 4% and 12% of girls have had some sort of sexual experience with a male relative, with 1 out of every hundred having some sort of sexual experience with a father or stepfather. Kinsey and colleagues (1953) reported a 5% incidence of incest in a nonclinical population.

Sibling incest, such as that between brothers and sisters, is believed to be even more widespread than incest that occurs between fathers or stepfathers and daughters (Cole, 1982; Finkelhor, 1978; Smith and Israel, 1987). A study with college students found that 15% of the females and 10% of the males had had some type of sexual experience with a sibling, but only 12% of them had ever disclosed the experience to anyone (Finkelhor, 1980).

Estimates of the incidence and prevalence of incest are likely underreported due to the secrecy of the behavior, the difficulties associated with its disclosure, and fear of the consequences that may result to the individuals involved and the family as a whole following its revelation (Matsakis, 1991). Sibling incest is believed to suffer from even greater underreporting than parent-child incest. First, there exists a perception that sibling incest is less traumatic than that effectuated by a parent or parent surrogate because it does not violate generational boundaries (Canavan, Meyer, and Higgs, 1992). Too, it may be more difficult to blame a child who initiates the sexual contact with a sibling than it is to blame an adult. It is commonly believed that mutual sexual exploration by children of similar age constitutes a normal event in the children's psychosocial development (Canavan, Meyer, and Higgs, 1992).

The extent to which statistics reflect delayed reporting is also unclear. Critics of delayed disclosures of childhood incest have claimed that many of the reports may be false and reflect distorted and inaccurate memories of childhood events (Doe, 1991). However, several studies suggest that forgetting abuse intermittently or for varying periods of time may not be uncommon (Briere and Conte, 1993; Cameron, 1994; Herman and Shatzow, 1987; Loftus, 1993; Roesler and Wind, 1994; Williams, 1994). Forgetting abuse appears to be more likely if the abuse occurred at a young age, if it was repeated, if the child feared death following the disclosure of the abuse, if there was physical injury associated with the sexual abuse, if the abuse involved multiple persons, and if there were relatively more psychiatric symptoms present (Briere and Conte, 1993). It has been hypothesized that repressed memory may result from dissociation, which acts as a defensive disruption of awareness, identity, and memory in response to overwhelming trauma (Kihlstrom, 1994). It has also been suggested that traumatic memory may be encoded differently than normal memory and excluded from the verbal representational system, thereby forming the basis for flashbacks in affective or somatic modalities (Rothschild, 2000; van der Kolk, 1994).

The Etiology of Incestuous Sexual Behavior

Parent-Child Incestuous Behavior

Numerous theories have been advanced in an attempt to explain why a parent might choose to have sexual relations with his or her blood- or law-related child. These theories include mate deprivation, opportunism, the failure of an incest avoidance mechanism, psychopathy, and a preference for sexually immature children.

The theory of mate deprivation posits that men who are deprived of sexual partners of their preferred age and gender will target individuals from the next most preferred category (Quinsey, 1977, 1986). The theory of opportunism is somewhat analogous to that of mate deprivation. This theory hypothesizes that normal men may exhibit interest in sexually immature girls (Hall, Hirschman, and Oliver, 1995; Harris, Rice, Quinsey, and Chaplin, 1996) and may engage in sexual activity with such a person if one is available, is somewhat sexually attractive, and is not resistant (Rice and Harris, 2002). Empirical research lends some support to the idea that a not insubstantial proportion of men may be sexually interested in children. Briere and Runtz (1989) reported from a study of college men that 21% experienced sexual attraction to small children, 9% acknowledged having fantasies of sex with a child, 5% had masturbated to fantasies of sex with a child, and 7% indicated some likelihood of having sex with a child.

The incest avoidance mechanism derives from a selectionist perspective. As implied by inclusive fitness theory (Daly and Wilson, 1988), mechanisms exist to inhibit inbreeding, which increases the expression of recessive genes. Accordingly, the descendants of individuals who have sexual intercourse with their close relatives are less successful reproductively (Thornhill, 1991; Van den Berghe, 1983). The Westermarck hypothesis posits that individuals who are reared together from childhood have an aversion to having sexual intercourse with each other (Shepher, 1983; Westermarck, 1891). A similar mechanism may operate through the caretaking of young children to discourage parental sexual relations with their children (Williams and Finkelhor, 1995). Such close attachments are believed to minimize the likelihood of incest, while weaker familial bonds and access may increase the likelihood of its occurrence (Maletzky, 1996).

A number of studies appear to support these hypotheses. Biological fathers who committed incest have been found to be less involved in child care activities as compared with nonincestuous fathers (Parker and Parker, 1986; Williams and Finkelhor, 1995). Having a stepfather appears to increase a girl's risk of being sexually abused (Finkelhor, Hotaling, Lewis, and Smith, 1990). Compared to nonincestuous men having sexual encounters with children, incestuous biological fathers appear to have relatively less interest in children generally (Seto, Lalumière, and Kunban, 1999).

Mental illness and psychopathy have also been suggested as a possible explanation for parent-child incest (Rice and Harris, 2002). One group of researchers concluded from their investigations of father-daughter incest where the daughter was under the age of 12 that the fathers had a "pathological obsession with sex" (Gebhard, 1965: 227). Although a number of studies have failed to confirm the existence of psychosis prior to the occurrence of the incest (Cavallin, 1966; Lukianowicz, 1972; Weiner, 1962), others have noted that a small proportion of the incestuous fathers in their samples evidenced psychosis (Medlicott, 1967; Merland, Fiornetini, and Orsini, 1962). Kubo (1959) reported from his investigation that cases of incest occurring among urban, middle-class families appeared to involve psychosis, unlike those found among rural families of lower socioeconomic status. These findings have been interpreted as suggesting that the subcultural context may be important in permitting the overt occurrence of incest (Meiselman, 1978). However, they may also reflect investigator bias relating to behavioral expectations of individuals within various socioeconomic strata which may, in turn, be reflective of cultural biases. Still other researchers have noted the offender's development of psychosis after the occurrence of the incest (Cavallin, 1966; Weinberg, 1955) and the paranoid tendencies among incestuous fathers, even in the absence of psychosis (Cavallin, 1966; Raphling, Carpenter and Davis, 1967; Weiner, 1962). Pedophiles are believed to constitute a distinct group of offenders; pedophilia is addressed below.

Meiselman (1978) has suggested from her review of the literature that various forms of paternal dysfunction may provide the basis for the initiation of incestuous relations. Paternal dysfunction may manifest as psychopathy, psychosis, drunkenness, pedophilia, mental defect, or reaction to stress. In addition, she hypothesized that some fathers exhibit endogamic traits, defined as a heavy dependence on family members fo the satisfaction of emotional and sexual needs and an inability or unwillingness to satisfy sexual needs outside of the family, accompanied by the existence of either a personality disorder or a subcultural milieu that tolerates incest.

Maternal circumstances have also been implicated in the occurrence of father-child incest, including a weak incest taboo due to the mother's own experiences with incest in her birth family (Raphling, Carpenter, and Davis, 1967) and the existence of a serious illness that results in maternal absence from the home or incapacitation and consequent unavailability (Kubo, 1959; Maisch, 1972; Weinberg, 1955). The mothers of daughters who were the object of incestuous relations have also been characterized as passive and dependent (Kaufman, Peck, and Taiguri, 1954; Weinberg,

1955), masochistic in the sense of embracing martyrdom (Meiselman, 1978), "promiscuous" outside of the marriage as the result of extreme emotional dependence on men (Meiselman, 1978), or averse to sexual relations (Cormier, Kennedy, and Sangowicz, 1962; Maisch, 1972).

Sibling Incestuous Behavior

Sibling incest has been explained as a response to a pervasive experience of powerlessness:

Children may turn to each other for [emotional] warmth, while others in a dominant position, such as older brothers and sisters, may forcibly take from younger siblings what is not being given to them voluntarily. A weaker sibling may not be much of a conquest, but at least the need to express power over something in their lives is temporarily satisfied (Renvoizé, 1982: 138).

Researchers have identified two major types of sibling incest. Nurturance-related relationships are premised on mutuality, loyalty, and compassion. They are often entered into as a means of protection from an abusive or neglectful family environment. As such, they may offer "safe haven" from the family dynamics, but may also inhibit individual development (Bank and Kahn, 1982).

In contrast, power-oriented incestuous sibling relationships often involve violence and victimization. One researcher has delineated three subtypes of victimization: victimization may be of a younger, naïve sister, who is used for sexual experimentation by her older brother; of a younger sister by an outcast brother who uses her as a substitute for female peers; or acts by an older abused brother who utilizes violence and coercion (Courtois, 1988). This schema of victimization and violence clearly ignores instances of incestuous conduct initiated by female with their male siblings or that between same-sex siblings.

It has also been suggested that older brother-younger sister incest results from unresolved Oedipal issues in both siblings and that its expression will not result in harm to the sister (Arnst and Ladd, 1981; Lukjanowicz, 1972). Other researchers have disputed the resulting lack of harm, pointing to the occurrence of diverse sequelae: lowered self-esteem (Finkelhor, 1980), fear of sexual assault and sexual difficulties in relationships (Cole, 1982; Meiselman, 1978, 1980; Russell, 1986), depression and guilt concerning the activity (Cole, 1982), low self-esteem and repeated victimization (De Young, 1982), and somatization, suicide, and substance use (Cole, 1982).

Pedophilia and Child Molestation

Defining Terms

Significant confusion surrounds the use of the term "pedophilia." First, the term pedophilia is often used to refer to incest, in addition to nonfamilial adult-child sexual relations (e.g., McConaghy, 2001). In addition, the term "pedophilia" has been used by a number of researchers to encompass a much broader population. Finkelhor and Araji (1986), for example, have used the term to refer to all individuals who have any sexual interest or contact with a child, regardless of the transient nature of that interest:

Specifically, we define pedophilia as occurring when an adult has a conscious sexual interest in prepubertal children. We infer that sexual interest from one of two behaviors: either (a) the adult has had some sexual contact with a child (meaning that he touched the child or had the child touch him with the purpose of becoming sexually aroused), or (b) the adult has masturbated to sexual fantasies involving children (Finkelhor and Araji, 1986: 146-147).

Yet another researcher has said of pedophilia and pedophiliac relationships:

Pedophiliac relationships can be very diverse. They have their own dynamics, are not always monogamous, and although the duration can be quite lengthy, are by definition limited to the youth of the younger partner . . . There are pedophiliac relationships without sexual contact, and there can also be single pedosexual contacts without a relationship. Furthermore, pedophiliac feelings do not necessarily play a part in every case of sexual contact with a child (Sandfort, 1984: 124).

These uses of the term pedophilia are in contrast to its use as a clinical diagnosis. The *Diagnostic and Statistical Manual, Fourth Edition, Text Revision* requires that three elements be present to warrant a diagnosis of pedophilia: (1) recurrent and intense sexually arousing fantasies, sexual urges, or behaviors involving sexual activity with a prepubescent child or children for a period of at least six months; (2) marked distress or interpersonal difficulties as a result of these urges or fantasies, or actually having acted on them; and (3) the individual is at least 16 years of age and at least five years older than the children who are the subject of the urges, fantasies, or behavior (American Psychiatric Association, 2000). However, individuals who are in late adolescence and are involved in a sexual relationship with someone who is 12 or 13 years of age will not be considered to be suffering from pedophilia. Underlying this definition and these criteria is an implicit characterization of pedophilia as an illness.

Additional confusion results from the use of terms that may or may not be used synonymously. For instance, although the term "child molester" has been equated with pedophile, at least some authors have distinguished between the two concepts. Others have equated child molestation with child sexual abuse and a child molester with a sexual abuser (e.g., Murray, 2000). Depending upon the term used, the focus appears to be either on the adult (pedophile, sexual abuser, child molester) or the age of the child and the act (child sexual abuse, child molestation), but none of the terms used encompass the totality of the circumstances.

Perspectives on Nonfamilial Adult-Child Sexual Activity

Although child-adult sexual behavior is now considered to be at times an illness and often a criminal activity that is regulated through our criminal codes, history indicates that at one time, sexual relations between prepubescent children and adults were considered acceptable. In England, the legal age of consent for girls for sex and for marriage was set at 12 until 1929. In the United States, it was set at 14 in many jurisdictions until relatively recently (Bullough, 1990). As of 1997, the age of consent continued to be set at 12 for heterosexual activity in New Zealand, and for both heterosexual and homosexual activity in the Netherlands, Spain, and Malta. The age of 15 prevailed in the Czech Republic, Denmark, Greece, France, Poland, and Sweden (Royal Commission into the New South Wales Police Service, 1997).

Empirical research is often based on cases that have been presented for criminal prosecution, resulting in samples that may represent the most egregious instances of adult-child sexual behavior or instances that are most susceptible to discovery. A review of 511 cases of sexual abuse of children ages 2 months to 12 years of age in Montreal found that the majority of the children were girls (Dube and Hebert, 1988). In more than three-quarters of the cases, the child knew the adult and the sexual activity occurred only once. School-aged children were more likely to be the sexual target of someone outside of the family, while male children were more likely to be assaulted by strangers and to suffer more severe injury.

It is of note that at least a proportion of men who engage in sex with children do not distinguish in terms of sex. In an interview-based study with 561 men who were seeking evaluation and/or treatment for a paraphilia, it was found that, of all of the men who had been involved in non-incestuous female pedophilia, 35% were also involved in non-incestuous male pedophilia, 35% in incestuous female pedophilia, and 12% in incestuous male pedophilia

(Abel, Becker, Cunningham-Rathner, Mittelman, and Rouleau, 1988).

Various theories have been proffered to explain why adults might become sexually involved with children. Finkelhor and Araji (1986) have classified the various theories that have been developed to explain pedophilia into four categories: (1) those that explain why an individual might engage in or fantasize about sexual relations with a child (emotional congruence); (2) theories that focus on how individuals could become sexually aroused by a child (sexual arousal to children); (3) theories that focus on why individuals are unable to obtain sexual and emotional satisfaction from other sources (blockage); and (4) explanations of why individuals are not deterred by social conventions from their behavior (disinhibition).

It has been postulated that inappropriate sexual arousal may underlie adults' sexual interest in children. However, research indicates that in a large proportion of cases, sexual activity with a child occurs only once and appears to be opportunistic rather than indicative of a continuing motivation or a pattern of behavior (Finkelhor, Williams, and Burns, 1989).

Pedophilia has also been attributed to the lack of adequate emotional and sexual gratification, leading to the choice of children as an outlet (Freund, Langevin, and Cibiri, 1972). Empirical data exist that both support and refute this theory. Although some pedophiles have been shown to be shy and passive (Ames and Hovston, 1990) and lacking in social skills (Oberholser and Beck, 1986), research also indicates that pedophiles may marry and father children (Finkelhor, Williams, and Burns, 1989).

Yet another theory postulates that pedophiles are disinhibited through the use of alcohol (Araji and Finkelhor, 1985). A study of 203 inmates in a state hospital who had been convicted of child molestation found that almost one-half of them had been drinking prior to their sexual activity with a child, and almost one-third had been heavily drinking (Rada, 1976). This theory fails, however, to explain why half of the inmates who had not been drinking performed sex acts with a child.

It has also been hypothesized that sexual abusers of children were themselves sexually abused as children (Greenberg, Bradford, and Curry, 1993). A study based on self-reports of 344 men concluded that some of those classified as pedophiles had, indeed, experienced sexual abuse as children (Freund, Watson, and Dickey, 1990).

Child Marriage

Background

Child marriage continues to this day, both in the United States and in other countries despite a 2001 declaration by the United Nations Children Fund characterizing the marriage of children under the age of 18 as a human rights violation (Anon., 2003). In Alabama, children can marry at the age of 14, with parental consent (Tolkinnen, 2003). In Utah, a 16-year old alleged that she had been whipped for refusing to marry her uncle, with whom her family had arranged her marriage (Carter, 1998; Rivera, 1998). Romanian officials initiated an investigation into the forced marriage of a 12-year old girl with a 15-year old boy that had been arranged by their parents (Associated Press, 2003). In India, despite a decline in frequency, child marriage continues, justified as a religious sacrament under Hindu law (Nagi, 1993; Nagpaul, 1988); in the state of Rajasthan, more than one-half of all marriages occur before the girl has reached the age of 15 (United Nations Children's Fund, 2001). In Niger, a study conducted through UNICEF found that almost one-half of women ages 20 to 24 were married before they had reached their fifteenth birthday (United Nations Children's Fund, 2001).

It has been argued that parents arrange marriages for their young girls for either or both of two reasons. First, girls may be considered to be less valuable than boys because they will ultimately leave home and will not contribute to the household income or support their parents as they age. Consequently, it is argued, the bride-price that will be received in exchange for her hand in marriage will help to support her family, pay off its debts, and provide funds for the purchase of her brothers' brides (Forum on Marriage and the Rights of Women and Girls, 2000; Warner, 2004). Second, it is argued, an early marriage assures the girl's virginity at the time of marriage and protects her from sexual predators and the risk of illegitimate pregnancy, which would decrease her value (Forum on Marriage and the Rights of Women and Girls, 2000; Warner, 2004).

Less cynically, parents may recognize the limited range of options available to their female offspring, who may have been raised in poverty, with limited educational and employment opportunities available. Marriage may realistically provide the only option for a somewhat secure economic future. In addition, some parents may believe that the arranged marriage of their daughter will fulfill a religious obligation (Nagi, 1993).

The Legal Context

Various international conventions contain provisions that seemingly place establish parameters for marriage. These provisions are summarized in Table 2, below.

Despite these provisions, child marriage is permitted and continues in many countries. First, the provisions are not self-executing; compliance requires that each State Party to the convention develop mechanisms for their implementation and enforcement. The United States, for instance, has not ratified either the Convention on the Rights of the Child or the Convention on the Right to Consent to Marriage, Minimum Age for Marriage and Registration of Marriages (Warner, 2004). Second, nations have the ability to file a reservation with respect to specific provisions. For example, Egypt formulated the following reservation to the

Table 2. International Conventions with Provisions Arguably Limiting Child Marriage

Convention	Provision
African Charter	Article 21(2): "Child marriage and the betrothal of girls and boys shall be prohibited, and effective action including legislation shall betaken to specify the minimum age of marriage to be eighteen years."
Convention on Consent to Marriage, Minimum Age for Marriage and Registration of Marriages	Article 1.1: No marriage shall be legally entered into without the full and free consent of both parties, such consent to be expressed by them in person after due publicity and in the presence of the authority competent to solemnize the marriage and of witnesses, as prescribed by law.
Convention on the Elimination of All Forms of Discrimination Against Women	Article 16.1: provides for full equality between men and women on the right to enter freely into marriage, the right to select a spouse, and the right to enter marriage with free and full consent
Convention on the Rights of the Child	Article 1: A child means every human being below the age of eighteen years, unless under the law applicable to the child, majority is attained earlier. Article 3: "in all actions concerning children . . . the best interests of the child shall be a primary consideration" Article 24.3: States Parties are to abolish "traditional practices prejudicial to the health of children."

Continued

Table 2. (*Continued*)

Convention	Provision
Convention Against Torture, and Other Cruel, Inhuman or Degrading Treatment or Punishment	Torture is defined as: an act by which severe pain or suffering, whether physical or mental, is intentionally inflicted on a person . . . for any reason based on discrimination of any kind, when such pain or suffering is inflicted by or at the instigation of or with the consent or acquiescence of a public official or other person acting in an official capacity."
Supplementary Convention on the Abolition of Slavery, the Slave Trade, and Institutions and Practices Similar to Slavery	States Parties are to take all action to eliminate "any institution or practice whereby . . . [a] woman, without the right to refuse, is promised or given in marriage on the payment of consideration in money or in kind to her parents, guardian, family or any other person or group."
United Nations' Protocol to Prevent, Suppress, and Punish Trafficking in Persons, Especially Women and Children	the recruitment, transportation, transfer, harbouring or receipt of persons, by means of the threat or use of force or other forms of coercion, of abduction, of fraud, of deception, of the abuse of power or of a position of vulnerability . . . or of the giving or receiving of payments or benefits to achieve the consent of a person having control over another person, for the purpose of exploitation. Exploitation shall include, at a minimum, the exploitation of the prostitution of others or other forms of sexual exploitation . . . forced labour or services, slavery or practices similar to slavery, servitude, or the removal of organs (United Nations Office for Drug Control and Crime Prevention, 2000).

Table 2. (*Continued*)

Convention	Provision
U.S. President's Interagency Council on Women	All acts involved in the recruitment, transport, harboring or sale of persons within national or across international borders through deception or fraud, coercion or force, or debt bondage for purposes of placing persons in situations of forced labor or services, such as forced prostitution or sexual services, domestic servitude, or other forms of slavery-like practices

Convention on the Elimination of All Forms of Discrimination Against Women:

Reservation to the text of article 16 concerning the equality of men and women in all matters relating to marriage and family relations during marriage and upon its dissolution, without prejudice to the Islamic Sharia's provisions whereby women are accorded rights equivalent to those of the spouses so as to ensure a just balance between them. This is out of respect for the sacrosanct nature of the firm religious beliefs which govern marital relations in Egypt and which may not be called into question and in view of the fact that one of the most important bases of those relations is an equivalency of rights and duties so as to ensure complementary [sic] which guarantees true equality between the spouses. The provisions of the Sharia lay down that the husband shall pay bridal money to the wife and maintain her fully and shall also make a payment to her upon divorce, whereas the wife retains full rights over her property and is not obliged to spend anything on her keep. The Sharia therefore restricts the wife's rights to divorce by making it contingent on a judge's ruling, whereas no such restriction is laid down in the case of the husband (Convention on the Elimination of All Forms of Discrimination Against Women, 1979).

Third, a number of countries provide in their domestic law that an individual attains the age of majority upon marriage, so that he or she is no longer considered a child; this essentially eliminates any protections provided by the Convention on the Rights of the Child (Population Council, 2004).

Relatively little empirical research has been conducted on recently-occurring child marriages. A study by Nagi (1993) of child marriages among 200 families in four villages in the Indian state of Rajasthan found that boys below the age of 11 were married in 23% of the families, while girls below the age of 11 were married in 51% of the families. More than three-quarters of married female members were married before they attained the age of 15. The incidence of child marriage was found to be higher in families with a lower income, those with little or no contact with urban life such as through employment, and those in which the head of the household was illiterate (Nagy, 1993).

Child Partnering and Health

Family Relations and Incest

There has been a tendency, reflected in large part in both our legal and clinical perspectives on incest, to view incest as a discrete event of sexual intercourse among family members, to decontextualize "the act," to view the act itself as "the problem," and to attribute blame as a means of situating incest-related guilt in a specified individual (Reidy and Hochstadt, 1993; Taubman, 1984). Mothers may often be blamed for their failure to detect and/or report the incest, while daughters may be accused of causing the incest through their alleged seductive behavior (McIntyre, 1981). Incestuous events may be attributed to the existence of hostility between a mother and her daughter, as well as role reversal between the two. Among mental health professionals, the degree to which the father is blamed has been found to be inversely related to the age of the child, with increasing blame assigned to the father with the child's younger age (Kalichman, Craig, and Crowe, 1986). Male, as contrasted with female, clinicians, appear to attribute greater blame to the mother and daughter in cases of father-daughter incest, regardless of the age of the daughter. A study conducted with teachers and social workers found that the level of a child's resistance and the extent of an adolescent victim's prior sexual experience have an important impact on the attribution of blame to a specified individual (Johnson, Owens, Dewey, and Eisenberg, 1990).

The importance of focusing on the family dynamic, and not only the adult and the child involved, is underscored by research findings related to disclosures of incest. A study by Everson and colleagues (1989) found that less than one-half of the mothers of 88 child victims of intrafamilial sexual abuse were consistently supportive of their children following the disclosure of the incest. Many of the women experienced extreme anguish and intense role conflict between their responsibilities and commitment as a parent and their allegiance to their partner. A study by Burgess and colleagues (1977) of 44 cases of incest found that families identified divided loyalty between the abusers and the victims as the major issue. Nineteen of the cases had involved biological fathers or stepfathers. In yet another study of 43 mothers, it was found that more than one-half believed their daughters, while others were protective of their partners and ambivalent about their children (Browning and Boatman, 1977). Mothers have been found to be more likely to believe the child's report of the incest if the offender is an extended family members, such as a grandfather, uncle or cousin; if the nature of the contact was oral- or digital-genital or –anal, rather than genital-genital; and if the mother was outside of the home when the sexual encounters occurred (Sirles and Franke, 1989). These findings highlight the extent to which incest affects members of the family in addition to those engaged in "the act," and lend empirical support to family systems theorists, who perceive incest as a means of sustaining a dysfunctional family system (Sheinberg, 1992).

Unfortunately, a focus on the family context may evolve into a misplaced reliance on overly simplistic and stereotypical portrayals of the "incestuous family," which may be neither informative nor useful in specific circumstances: a family characterized by ill-defined boundaries, a father with damaged self-esteem and impulse control, a mother who is a silent partner, and a needy child who, in her search for affection, may be predisposed to incestuous assault (Carozza and Heirsteiner, 1982). Still other researchers view incest as one element in the use by families of silence or ineffectual communication to sustain a family system (Donalek, 2001).

Feminist theorists have viewed incest as a linear issue with the abuser having power and control over the victim, who has neither power nor control, thereby assigning blame to the perpetrator alone (Ehrmin, 1996). Indeed, the feminist perspective on incest asserts that the family therapy literature ignores the patriarchal context of incest and obscures its inherent gender politics (James and Mackinnon, 1990). Although this conceptual model acknowledges and incorporates the potential influence of the larger environment, which is absent from systems theory that focuses on the family system alone, it is itself deficient in its failure to adequately encompass and explain incestuous behavior of adult females initiated with male or female children, and that of adult males with male children.

Incest, however, may also be conceived of as a process that is situated within a societal, familial, and individual context, that is, an interactive, multisystemic context. A society may, for instance, be patriarchal, may depersonalize and objectify both men and women in their ascribed roles, and may emphasize economic productivity as a measure of an individual's true value (Taubman, 1984). It has also been argued that U.S. society has sexualized children and simultaneously denies that it has done so (Kincaid, 1998). Various depictions of children have been proffered to substantiate this assertion: the beauty contests for little girls, who are dressed and made up to look older and sexier; marketing strategies—successful, at that—that feature young boys and girls in sexually suggestive poses, such as Brooke Shields' "There is nothing between me and my jeans;" and the cinematic portrayal of sexualized youngsters, as in *Pretty Baby* (1978) and *The Teacher* (1974) (Kincaid, 1998).

The family context may encompass parental separation, partner abuse, diminished interest in sex, mental illness, substance use, and/or power conflicts. To some extent, however, the family system has been viewed as a separate entity, distinct and apart from the larger environmental context (Eist and Mandel, 1968; Haley, 1967; Machotka, Pittman, and Flomenhaft, 1967). It has been argued that an examination of the interaction of the family system with that of the community may be critical to effectuating a metamorphosis in the family dynamic (Alexander, 1985). The larger environment may become involved through referral to the health care, welfare, law enforcement, and/or judicial systems. Additionally, the nature of the family's interaction with the environmental system, such as an absence of information exchange, may have contributed to the development of an atmosphere that permitted the incestuous process to occur (Alexander, 1985). Unfortunately, relatively little research has focused on the aftermath of incest disclosure on individual family members and the family as an entity functioning as a system within the interplay of larger systems.

Child Development

Incest

Women who as children were the targets of father-child incest have reported that as children they experienced feelings of isolation; anticipation of additional abuse; fears of being killed, of being exposed as stigmatized, and of being tainted by the abuse; the use of resistance and/or fantasy in an attempt to escape what was happening; confusion about the meaning and the importance of the abuse; and anxiety about the need to keep the incest a secret and the need to protect their mothers and keep their parents' relationship together (Donalek, 2001). Adult women have also reported that as children they felt that they inhabited two worlds, one of abuse and one of normal family life (Donalek, 2001).

Silverman's (2001) account of her father's sexual behavior with her as a child poignantly relates these feelings and the difficulties that she experienced as a result. During her young childhood, the bath and nighttime rituals often included some form of genital contact. Silverman recounted her confusion, fear, and anxiety:

I am addicted to these terrifying new things. Addicted to terror. For terror, feel love. With terror, my body feels loved. Terror is the definition of love, a synonym proving love's existence. So I stubbornly sit in this house in order to enable my parents to love me. I need for my father to love me. And I believe that he does (Silverman, 2001:25).

Few researchers have examined the effects of incest on the development of young boys. Nasjleti (1980) reported from her review of effects that young boys who suffered incest were likely to fear being branded as sissies or homosexuals, becoming homosexual, or having their masculinity being called into question due to their failure to prevent an assault by a female. They were also concerned that they might be mentally ill because they had sex with their mothers and experienced feelings of shame due to their inability to protect themselves from a female.

Levels of maternal support appear to be more strongly predictive of a child's psychological functioning than either the type or the length of the abuse or the perpetrator's relationship to the child (Everson et al., 1989). Khan's (1963: 46-47) concept of "cumulative trauma" explains why the mother's response may be so critical:

[C]umulative trauma is a result of the breaches in the mother's role as a protective shield over the whole course of the child's development, from infancy to adolescence—that is to say, in all those areas of experience where the child continues to need the mother as an auxiliary ego to support his immature and unstable ego-functions . . . these breaches over the course of time and through the developmental process cumulate silently and invisibly . . . .

The mother's inability to adequately shield the child has been variously attributed to her own psychopathology, a loss or separation of the child from the mother, a handicap of the mother or sever illness of the child that create an impossible demand (Winnicott, 1952). The mother's continuing failure or inability to address the infant's needs adequately has been posited to result in adverse consequences to the infant's development, such as an excessive preoccupation by the child with the mother's needs (Winnicott, 1958).

Nonfamilial Adult-Child Sexual Interaction

It is often difficult to distinguish research findings pertaining to nonfamilial adult-child sexual interactions from those pertaining to incestuous relationships, because the two are often combined in the same studies. Additionally, variations in definitions, sampling strategies, study aims, and study design reduce comparability across studies.

Studies that have compared sexually abused children with those that have not been sexually abused have found that they may be more likely to engage in inappropriate sexual behavior, such as inappropriate sexual overtures towards other children or adults, and may have an earlier age of onset of sexual activity (Kendall-Tackett, Williams, and Finkelhor, 1993). In addition, they may be more likely to experience fear, nightmares, withdrawn behavior, symptoms of posttraumatic stress disorder, cruelty, delinquency, and self-injurious behavior (Kendall-Tackett, Williams, and Finkelhor, 1993). They may also be more likely to display high levels of dissociation, resulting in a disturbance in the integrative functions of memory and identity (Trickett and Putnam, 1993).

In contrast, it was reported from an interview-based study of 25 boys between the ages of 10 and 16 years of age who were involved in pedophiliac relationships with older men in the Netherlands that most of the boys characterized their sexual contacts with the adult men as predominately positive, that there appeared to be no negative influence on the boys' general sense of well-being, and the boys did not perceive these contacts as a misuse of authority by the adult (Sandfort, 1984). It was found that many of the boys had taken the initiative to establish *nonsexual* bonds with the adults. The researcher concluded that the desires of the boys played a key part in the relationship dynamic. Significant questions remain unanswered, however. For instance, although the boys characterized the dynamic as primarily a positive one, it may be possible that they did not have the experience or maturity to recognize abuse. This would be analogous to a woman who is in an abusive relationship who recognizes the abuse only after it has become increasingly severe and repetitive.

Women's Health

Mental Health

A history of incest has been found to be associated with later self-mutilation. The prevalence of self-mutilating behavior among individuals who were victims of incest as children has been found to range from 17% (Briere and Zaidi, 1989) to 58% (de Young, 1982). Research indicates that, compared to whites with histories of incest, women of color with such histories are less likely to self-mutilate (Turell and Armsworth, 2000), although the reasons for this difference remain unclear. The likelihood of self-mutilation appears to increase with increased duration and severity of the incest and initiation of the incest at a younger age. Women with incest histories who self-mutilate also appear, in comparison with their counterparts who do not self-mutilate, to have internalized messages of humiliation, shame, punishment for exhibiting emotions, and feelings of abandonment and isolation, leading some researchers to hypothesize that it is the idiosyncratic meaning attributed to the events by the individual that determines the likelihood of trauma, rather than the specific facts of the events (Turell and Armsworth, 2000). However, even among women with histories of incest who have diagnoses of posttraumatic stress disorder, it is a minority who engage in self-mutilation (Albach and Everaerd, 1992).

Not surprisingly, women with histories of incest may experience posttraumatic stress disorder following the incest (Coons, Cole, Pellow, and Milstein, 1990; Graziano, 1992). According to the *Diagnostic and Statistical Manual Fourth Edition, Text Revision*, used to diagnose mental disorders, posttraumatic stress disorder may result when an individual both (1) witnesses, experiences, or confronts an event or events that involve actual or threatened death, serious injury, or a threat to his or her integrity or the integrity of others, and (2) the person responds with intense fear, helplessness, or horror. To be diagnosed with the disorder, an individual must re-experience the traumatic event in at least one of four ways: (1) recurrent and intrusive distressing memories of the event, (2) recurring dreams of the event, (3) acting or feeling as if the event were recurring; (4) intense psychological distress following exposure to reminders of an aspect of the traumatic event, or (5) a physiological reaction to exposure to cues that symbolize or resemble an aspect of the event (American Psychiatric Association, 2000). Silverman described the "body memories" that she experienced in response to external events that prompted memories of the prolonged father-daughter incest:

Without warning, my legs feel paralyzed. I wake up in the middle of the night and feel that my hair is being pulled, pulling my head back and back until I can barely swallow. My head feels as if it's severed from my throat (Silverman, 2001: 202).

Diagnosis further requires that the individual persistently avoid stimuli associated with the trauma and experience a general numbing of responsiveness that did not exist prior to the event. This avoidance must be manifested by three or more of the following: (1) attempts to avoid feelings, thoughts, or conversations associated with the traumatic event(s), (2) attempts to avoid people, places, or activities that engender memories of the trauma, (3) inability to remember an important aspect of the trauma, (4) significantly reduced interest or participation in important activities, (5) a feeling of detachment or estrangement from others, (6) a restricted range of affect, and (7) a feeling that the future or life events will somehow be shortened or abbreviated. A person suffering from this disorder must also be found to be experiencing two or more of the following symptoms: sleep disturbances, irritability or outbursts of anger, difficulty concentrating, hypervigilance, and an exaggerated startle response. The diagnostic symptoms must be of at least one month's duration and cause clinically significant distress or impairment in social or occupational functioning or in some other arena of functioning (American Psychiatric Association, 2000).

The specific consequences of PTSD vary with the nature of the trauma, the age of the victim, the response to the trauma, and the level of support provided to the victim following the traumatic event(s) (Rothschild, 2000). In general, sequelae may include periods of overactivity that alternate with periods of exhaustion, panic at the appearance of reminders of the trauma, and a perception that many things in the environment are dangerous. As a result of these pervasive fears, sufferers of PTSD may eventually have very limited and isolated lives (Rothschild, 2000).

Substance use has been documented among some women with histories of incest (Riszt, 1979; Streicher-Bremer, 2001). Streicher-Bremer (2001) reported from her preliminary investigation of female heroin users with a history of incest that drugs were utilized as a means of escaping difficult and unpleasant feelings.

A history of incest has also been found to be associated with eating disorders. Silverman (2000: 193-194) described her own response to the incest that she experienced:

I have an eating disorder and a sexual addiction. With food, I'm mostly anorectic, addicted to starvation in order not to feel, to numb-out. I watch my body grow thinner than light. No one can touch it or see it. It's a gray wisp, barely visible, refracting particles of light . . . By starving, I believe I am strong, not weak. I am the only one who can control what I will eat. I am the only one who will control the fate of my body . . . I'm terrified of intimacy. To keep men from truly seeing me, from truly knowing me, all I speak are words of seduction, words my father taught me, words of emotional isolation.

Sexual Behavior and Functioning

Studies of women with histories of incest have often reported sexual promiscuity as one of the sequelae (e.g., Lukianoiwicz, 1972; Maisch, 1972; Medlicott, 1967; Riszt, 1979). The validity of these findings is uncertain in view of significant methodological problems associated with the conduct of the studies. Many of the studies suffered from selection bias as a result of their inclusion of only women drawn from clinical and forensic samples. Societal standards for female sexual behavior existing at the time the studies were conducted were significantly harsher than they might be today. Additionally, use of the term "promiscuous" to describe resulting behavior serves only to cast moral judgment, rather than to describe in a meaningful way the specific outcome, so that it is unclear what type or frequency of behavior is actually encompassed within that term.

A number of studies that have reported increased sexual activity among women with histories of incest indicate that the higher levels of sexual activity appear to occur during early adulthood and such periods appear to be transitory (Finkelhor, 1980; Herman, 1981; Meiselman, 1978). One survey of college students, for instance, found that the women with histories of sibling incest had higher levels of sexual activity than those without such histories, but the difference between these two groups dissipated as the women moved into adulthood (Finkelhor, 1980).

Sexual difficulties among women who experienced incest have been reported in many studies. These difficulties have included a fear of sex (Becker et al., 1982, 1984); a lack of sexual desire (Becker et al., 1982, 1984; Jackson et al., 1990; Westerlund, 1983); sexual nonresponsiveness (Jackson et al., 1990; Meiselman, 1978; Westerlund, 1983); orgasmic dysfunction, such as the ability to be orgasmic only with a new partner (Meiselman, 1978; Westerlund, 1983) or to be orgasmic in the absence of sexual desire or arousal (McGuire and Wagner, 1979; Westerlund, 1983); flashbacks during sexual activity (Becker et al., 1984; Herman, 1981; Meiselman, 1978; Westerlund, 1983); and complaints of vaginismus, dyspareunia, and/or pelvic pain (Becker et al., 1982, 1984; Caldirola et al., 1983; Jackson et al., 1990).

Relationships

Women with histories of incest have been found to have difficulty being emotionally close to others, poor self-esteem, and difficulties dealing with feelings of anger (Owens, 1984).

A number of studies have examined sexual orientation among women with incest histories. Many of the studies have reported that a proportion of the women who experienced incest had had same-sex sexual experiences and/or self-identified as lesbian (Finkelhor, 1980; Herman, 1981; Meiselman, 1978). Other studies of the histories of lesbians have found that a minority had suffered incest (Simari and Baskin, 1982). However, no causal link has been established between incest, whether same-sex or opposite-sex, and later sexual orientation or preference.

Implications for Research and Practice

Although there is some data to the contrary, available research clearly documents the ill-effects of child-adult sexual activity on the child, regardless of whether that activity occurs with a member of the child's family, a non-family member known to the child, or a stranger. However, our ability to utilize these data for prevention and intervention programs is hindered by the lack of consistency across studies in the definitions used and in the failure to distinguish the child-adult relationship and the context in which it occurs. For instance, are the psychological effects of familial sexual different in frequency or severity than those of nonfamilial sexual activity between an adult and child? Does sexual activity that consists of kissing only, or exposure of genitals without touching result in the same adverse health consequences as does penetration? The intervention approach to be taken in instances of adult-child incestuous activity may be vastly different than those that would be effective in the prevention of child marriage to older adults in communities where, even though illegal, the practice remains common and socially acceptable.

These differences may also have implications for the clinician. The resolution of one's experience as a child who has been the subject of sexual activity with an adult family member may be quite different than that of a child who was assaulted by a stranger. In the former instance, the child, or possibly the now-adult, may have an investment in continuing the family relationship, while in the latter, no such connection to the adult is contemplated. Clearly, attention must be focused on the entire family and not only on the child and the adult who engaged in the sexual activity.

References

Albach, F., Everaerd, W. (1992). Posttraumatic stress symptoms in victims of childhood incest. *Psychotherapy and Psychosomatics* 57: 143-151.

Alexander, P.C. (1985). A systems theory conceptualization of incest. *Family Process* 24: 79-88.

American Medical Association. (1985). Diagnostic and treatment guidelines concerning child abuse and neglect. *Journal of the American Medical Association* 254: 796-800.

American Psychiatric Association. (2000). *Diagnostic and Statistical Manual, Fourth Edition, Text Revision.* Washington, D.C.: American Psychiatric Association.

Ames, M.A., Hovston, D.A. (1990). Legal, social, and biological definitions of pedophilia. *Archives of Sexual Behavior* 19: 333-342.

Anon. (2003). Child Marriage: An Issue Whose Time Has Come?, Nov. 10. Available at http://www.nospank.net/boysandgirls.htm. Last accessed July 25, 2004.

Araji, S., Finkelhor, D. (1985). Explanations of pedophilia: Review of empirical research. *Bulletin of the American Academy of Psychiatry and Law* 13: 71-83.

Arndt, W.B., Ladd, B. (1981). Sibling incest as an index of Oedipal conflict. *Journal of Assessment* 45: 52-58.

Associated Press. (2003). Romanians probe 12-year old's marriage. Available at http://www.nospank.net/boysandgirls.htm. Last accessed July 25, 2004.

Bank, S.P., Kahn, M. (1982). *The Sibling Bond.* New York: Basic Books.

Becker, J., Skinner, L., Abel, G., Axelrod, R., Cichon, J. (1984). Sexual problems of sexual assault survivors. *Women and Health* 9: 5-20.

Becker, J., Skinner, L., Abel, G., Treacy, E. (1982). Incidence and types of sexual dysfunctions in rape and incest victims. *Journal of Sex and Marital Therapy* 8: 65-74.

Benedict, M.I., Paine, L.L., Paine, L.A., Brandt, D., Stallings, R. (1999). The association of childhood sexual abuse with depressive symptoms during pregnancy, and selected pregnancy outcomes. *Child Abuse & Neglect* 23(7): 659-670.

Briere, J., Conte, J. (1993). Self-reported amnesia for abuse in adults molested as children. *Journal of Traumatic Stress* 6: 21-31.

Briere, J., Runtz, M. (1989). University males' sexual interest in children: Predicting potential indices of "pedophilia" in a nonforensic sample. *Child Abuse & Neglect* 13: 65-75.

Briere, J., Zaidi, L. (1989). Sexual abuse histories and sequelae in female psychiatric emergency room patients. *American Journal of Psychiatry* 146: 1602-1606.

Browning, D., Boatman, B. (1977). Incest: Children at risk. *American Journal of Psychiatry* 134: 69-72.

Bullough, V.L. (1990). History in adult human sexual behavior with children and adolescents in Western societies. In J.R. Feierman (Ed.), *Paedophilia: Biosocial Dimensions* (pp. 69-90). New York: Springer-Verlag.

Burgess, A.W., Homstrom, L.L., McCausland, A. (1977). Child sexual assault by a family member: Decisions following disclosure. *Victimology* 2: 36-50.

Burton, K., Myers, W.C. (1992). Child sexual abuse and forensic psychiatry: Evolving and controversial issues. *Bulletin of the American Academy of Psychiatry and Law* 20: 439-453.

Caldirola, D., Gemperle, M.B., Guzinski, G.M., Gross, R.J., Doerr, H. (1983). Incest and pelvic pain: The social worker as part of a research team. *Health & Social Work* 8(4): 309-319.

California Family Code § 2200 (2004).

Cameron, C. (1994). Women survivors confronting their abusers: Issues, decisions and outcomes. *Journal of Child Sexual Abuse* 3: 7-35.

Canavan, M.M., Meyer, W.I. III, Higgs, D.C. (1992). The female experience of sibling incest. *Journal of Marital and Family Therapy* 18(2): 129-142.

Carballo-Diéguez, A., Dolezal, C. (1995). Association between history of childhood sexual abuse and adult HIV-risk sexual behavior in Puerto Rican men who have sex with men. *Child Abuse & Neglect* 19(5): 595-605.

Carozza, P.M., Heirsteiner, C.L. (1982). Young female incest victims in treatment: Stages of growth seen with a group art therapy model. *Clinical Social Work Journal* 10(3): 165-175.

Carter, M. (2003). 16-year-old allegedly whipped for rebelling against arranged marriage to her uncle—Utah Gov. in political minefield. Associated Press, August 2. Available at http://www.nospank. net/boysandgirls.htm. Last accessed July 25, 2004.

Cavallin, H. (1966). Incestuous fathers: A clinical report. *American Journal of Psychiatry.* 166, 1132-1138.

Code of Alabama § 13A-13-3 (2004).

Cole, E. (1982). Sibling incest: The myth of benign sibling incest. *Women and Therapy* 5: 79-89.

Convention on Consent to Marriage, Minimum Age for Marriage and registration of Marriages. (1962, Nov. 9). 521 U.N.T.S. 231.

Convention on the Elimination of All Forms of Discrimination Against Women. (1979, Dec. 18). 1249 U.N.T.S. 13, 19 I.L.M. 33 (1980). Available at http://www.untreaty.un.org/ENGLISH/bible/ englishinternetbible/partI/chapterIV/treaty10.asp.

Convention on the Rights of the Child. Opened for signature November 20, 1989, 28 I.L.M. 1456, 1577 U.N.T.S. 3.

Coons, P.M. Cole, C., Pellow, T.A., Milstein, V. (1990). Symptoms of posttraumatic stress and dissociation in women victims of abuse. In R.P. Kluft (Ed.), *Incest-related Syndromes of Adult Psychopathology* (pp. 205-225). Washington, D.C.: American Psychiatric Press.

Cormier, B.M., Kennedy, M., Sangowicz, J. (1962). Psychodynamics of father-daughter incest. *Canadian Psychiatric Association Journal* 7: 203-217.

Courtois, C.A. (1988). *Healing the Incest Wound.* New York: Norton.

Daly, M., Wilson, M. (1988). The Darwinian psychology of discriminative parental solicitude. *Nebraska Symposium on Motivation* 35: 199-244.

De Young, M. (1982). Self injurious behavior in incest victims: A research note. *Child Welfare* 61: 577-584.

De Young M. (1982). *The Sexual Victimization of Children.* London: McFarland & Co.

Doe, J. (1991). How could this happen? Coping with a false accusation of incest and rape. *Issues in Child Abuse Accusations* 3: 154-165.

Donalek, J.G. (2001). First incest disclosure. *Issues in Mental Health Nursing* 22: 573-591.

Dube, R., Hebert, M. (1988). Sexual abuse of children under 12 years of age: A review of 511 cases. *Child Abuse and Neglect* 12: 321-330.

Ehrmin, J.T. (1996). No more mother blaming: A feminist nursing perspective on the mother's role in father-daughter incest. *Archives of Psychiatric Nursing* 10: 252-260.

Eist, H.I., Mandel, A.Y. (1968). Family treatment of ongoing incest behavior. *Family Process* 7: 216-232.

Ellenson, G. (1986). Disturbances of perception in adult female incest survivors. *Social Casework* 67: 149-159.

Everson, M.D., Hunter, W.M., Runyon, D.K., Edelsohn, G.A., Coulter, M.L. (1989). Maternal support following disclosure of incest. *American Journal of Orthopsychiatry* 59(2): 197-207.

Finkelhor, D. (1978). Psychological, cultural, and family factors in incest and family sexual abuse. *Journal of Marriage and Family Counseling* 4: 41-49.

Finkelhor, D. (1980). Sex among siblings: A survey on prevalence, variety, and effect. *Archives of Sexual Behavior* 9: 171-194.

Finkelhor, D. (1979). *Sexually Abused Children.* New York: Free Press.

Finkelhor, D., Araji, S. (1986). Explanations of pedophilia: A four factor model. *Journal of Sex Research* 22(2): 145-161.

Finkelhor, D., Hotaling, G., Lewis, I.A., Smith, C. (1990). Sexual abuse in a national sample of adult men and women: Prevalence, characteristics, and risk factors. *Child Abuse & Neglect* 14: 19-28.

Finkelhor, D., Williams, L.M., Burns, N. (1989). *Sexual Abuse in Day Care.* Newbury Park, California: Sage.

Forum on Marriage and the Rights of Women and Girls. (2000, May). *Early Marriage: Whose Right to Choose?* Available at http://www.crin.org/docs/resources/publications/WhoseRighttoChoose.pdf. Last accessed May 24, 2004.

Freund, K., Watson, R., Dickey, R. (1990). Does sexual abuse in childhood cause pedophilia? An exploratory study. *Archives of Sexual Behavior* 19: 557-569.

Gebhard, P.H. (1965). *Sex Offenders: An Analysis of Types.* New York: Harper & Row.

Graziano, R. (1992). Treating women incest survivors: A bridge between "cumulative trauma" and "post-traumatic stress." *Social Work in Health Care* 17(1): 69-85.

Greenber, D.M., Bradford, J., Curry, S. (1993). A comparison of sexual victimizations in the childhoods of pedophiles and hebephiles. *Journal of Forensic Sciences* 38: 432-436.

Greenspan, E.L., Rosenberg, M. (2000). *Martin's Annual Criminal Code.* Aurora, Ontario, Canada: Canada Law Book.

Haley, I. (1967). Toward a theory of pathological systems/ In G. Zuk, I. Boszormenyi-Nagy (Eds.). *Family Therapy and Disturbed Families.* Palo Alto, California: Science and Behavior Books.

Hall, N.G.C., Hirschman, R., Oliver, L.L. (1995). Sexual arousal and arousability to pedophilic stimuli in a community sample of normal men. *Behavior Therapy* 26: 681-684.

Harris, G.T., Rice, M.E., Quinsey, V.L., Chaplin, T.C. (1996). Viewing time as a measure of sexual interest among child molesters and normal heterosexual men. *Behaviour Research and Therapy* 34: 389-394.

Héritier, F. (1999). *Two Sisters and Their Mother: An Anthropology of Incest.* (Trans. J. Herman). New York: Urzone, Inc.

Herman, J. (1981). *Father-Daughter Incest.* Cambridge, Massachusetts: Harvard University Press.

Herman, J.L., Stratzow, E. (1987). Recovery and verification of memories of childhood sexual trauma. *Psychoanalytic Psychology* 4: 1-14.

Jackson, J.L., Calhoun, K.S., Amick, A.E., Maddever, H.M., Habif, V.L. (1990). Young adult women who report childhood intrafamilial sexual abuse: Subsequent adjustment. *Archives of Sexual Behavior* 19(3): 211-221.

Jacobs, J.L. (1990). Reassessing mother blame in incest. *Signs: Journal of Women in Culture and Society* 15: 500-515.

James, K., Mackinnon, L. (1990). The "incestuous family" revisited: A critical analysis of family therapy myths. *Journal of Marital and Family Therapy* 16(1): 71-88.

Johnson, P.A., Owens, R.G., Dewey, M.E., Eisenberg, N.E. (1990). Professional attributions of censure in father-daughter incest. *Child Abuse & Neglect* 14: 419-428.

Kalichman, S.C., Craig, M.E., Crowe, C.M. (1986). Incestuous abuse: Licensed and nonlicensed clinicians' attitudes and reporting. Paper presented at the meeting of the American Psychological Association, Washington, D.C.

Kaufman, I., Peck, A.L., Tagiuri, C.K. (1954). The family constellation and overt incestuous relations between father and daughter. *American Journal of Orthopsychiatry* 24: 266-27.

Kendall-Tackett, K.A., Williams, L., Finkelhor, D. (1993). The impact of sexual abuse on children: A review and synthesis of recent empirical studies. *Psychological Bulletin* 113(1): 164-180.

Khan, M. (1963). The concept of cumulative trauma. In *The Privacy of the Self.* New York: International Universities Press, 1974.

Kihlstrom, J.F. (1994). One hundred years of hysteria. In S.J. Lynn and J.W. Rhue (Eds.). *Dissociation. Clinical and Theoretical Perspectives.* New York: Guilford.

Kincaid, J.R. (1998). *Erotic Innocence: The Culture of Child Molesting.* Durham, North Carolina: Duke University Press.

Kinsey, A., Pomeroy, W., Martin, C. et al. (1953). *Sexual Behavior in the Human Female.* Philadelphia, Pennsylvania: W.B. Saunders.

Kubo, S. (1959). Researches and studies on incest in Japan. *Hiroshima Journal of Medical Sciences* 8: 99-159.

Langan, P., Harlow, C. (1994). *Child Rape Victims, 1992.* Washington, D.C.: Bureau of Justice Statistics, United States Department of Justice.

Laviola, M. (1992). Effects of older brother-younger sister incest: A study of the dynamics of 17 cases. *Child Abuse & Neglect* 16: 409-421.

Loftus, E. (1993). The reality of repressed memories. *American Psychologist* 48: 518-537.

Logan, T.K., Walker, R., Cole, J., Leukefeld, C. (2002). Victimization and substance abuse among women: Contributing factors, interventions, and implications. *Review of General Psychology* 6(4): 325-397.

Lukjanowicz, N. (1972). Incest. *British Journal of Psychiatry* 120: 301-313.

Machotka, J., Pittman, F.S. III, Flomenhaft, K. Incest as a family affair. *Family Process* 6: 98-116.

Maisch, H. (1972). *Incest.* (C. Bearne, Trans.). New York: Stein & Day.

Maletzky, B.M. (1996). Evolution, psychopathology, and sexual offending: Aping our ancestors. *Aggression and Violent Behavior* 1(4): 369-373.

Matsakis, A. (1991). *When the Bough Breaks.* Oakland, California: New Harbinger Publications.

McConaghy, N. (2001). Paedophilia: A review of the evidence. *Australian and New Zealand Journal of Psychiatry* 32: 252-265.

McIntyre, K. (1981). Role of mothers in father-daughter incest: A feminist analysis. *Social Work* 26: 462-466.

Medlicott, R. (1967). Parent-child incest. *Australian and New Zealand Journal of Psychiatry*, 1, 180-187.

Meiselman, K. (1978). Personality characteristics of incest history psychotherapy patients: A research note. *Archives of Sexual Behavior* 9: 195-197.

Meiselman, K.C. (1978). *Incest: A Psychological Study of Causes and Effects with Treatment Recommendations.* San Francisco: Jossey-Bass Publishers.

Merland, A., Fiorentini, H., Orsini, J. (1962). A propos de 34 expertises psychiatriques se rapportant a des actes d'inceste père-fille" [Concerning 34 psychiatric cases reported involving acts of father-daughter incest] *Annales de Médecine Legale* 42: 353-359.

Mollon, P. (1996). Incest, false accusations of incest and false denials of incest. *Journal of Mental Health* 5(2): 167-172.

Murray, J.B. (2000). Psychological profile of pedophiles and child molesters. *Journal of Psychology* 134(2): 211-224.

Nagi, B.S. (1993). *Child Marriage in India.* New Delhi, India: Mittal Publications.

Nagpaul, H. (1988). Secularism in India: Unresolved conflicts and persistent problems. *Politics, Culture, and Society* 2(2): 201-216.

Nasjleti, M. (1980). Suffering in silence: The male incest victims. *Child Welfare* 59(5): 269-275.

National Center for Victims of Crimes and Crime Victims Research and Treatment Center. (1992). *Rape in America: A Report to the Nation*. Arlington, Virginia: Author.

Neal, K. (1991). Incestuous child sexual abuse. *School of Social Work Journal* 15(2): 11-21.

Noll, J.G., Trickett, P.K., Putnam, F.W. (2003). A prospective investigation of the impact of childhood sexual abuse on the development of sexuality. *Journal of Consulting & Clinical Psychology* 71(3): 575-586.

Oberholser, J.C., Beck, J. (1986). Multimethod assessment of rapists, child molesters, and three control groups on behavioral and psychological measures. *Journal of Consulting and Clinical Psychology* 54: 682-687.

Owens, T.H. (1984). Personality traits of female psychotherapy patients with a history of incest: A research note. *Journal of Personality Assessment* 48(6): 606-608.

Parker, H., Parker, S. (1986). Father-daughter sexual abuse: An emerging perspective. *American Journal of Orthopsychiatry* 56: 531-549.

Population Council. (2004). Transitions to Adulthood: Married Adolescents/First-Time Parents, Dec. 6. Available at http://www.popcouncil.org/ta/childmar.html. Last accessed March 29, 2005.

Rada, T. (1976). Alcoholism and the child molester. *Annals of the New York Academy of Sciences* 273: 492-496.

Raphling, D.L., Carpenter, B.L., Davis, A. (1967). Incest: A genealogical study. *Archives of General Psychiatry* 16: 505-511.

Reidy, T.J., Hochstadt, N.J. (1993). Attribution of blame in incest cases: A comparison of mental health professionals. *Child Abuse & Neglect* 17: 371-381.

Renvoizé, J. (1982). *Incest: A Family Pattern*. London: Routledge & Kegan Paul.

Rice, M.E., Harris, G.T. (2002). Men who molest their sexually immature daughters: Is a special explanation required? *Journal of Abnormal Psychology* 111(2): 329-339.

Riszt, K. (1979). Incest: Theoretical and clinical views. *American Journal of Orthopsychiatry* 49(4): 680-691.

Rivera, R. (1998). 16-year-old girl testifies of beating. *Salt Lake Tribune,* July 23.

Roesler TA, Wind TW. (1994). Telling the secret: Adult women describe their disclosure of incest. *Journal of Interpersonal Violence* 9: 327-338.

Rothschild, B. (2000). *The Body Remembers: The Psychophysiology of Trauma and Trauma Treatment.* New York: W.W. Norton & Company.

Royal Commission into the New South Wales Police Service. (1997). *Final Report, Volume VI: The Paedophile Inquiry.* Sydney, Australia: Government of the State of New South Wales.

Rudd, J.M., Herzberger, S.D. (1999). Brother-sister incest—Father-daughter incest: A comparison of characteristics and consequences. *Child Abuse & Neglect* 23(9): 915-928.

Russell, D.E.H. (1983). The incidence and prevalence of intrafamilial and extrafamilial sexual abuse of female children. *Child Abuse & Neglect* 7: 133-146.

Russell, D.E.H. (1986). *The Secret Trauma: Incest in the Lives of Girls and Women.* New York: Basic Books.

Sandfort, T.G.M. (1984). Sex in pedophiliac relationships: An empirical investigation among a nonrepresentative group of boys. *Journal of Sex Research* 20(2): 123-142.

Schetky, D.H. (1990). A review of the literature on the long-term effects of childhood sexual abuse. In R.P. Kluft (Ed.), *Incest-related Syndromes of Adult Psychopathology* (pp. 35-54). Washington, D.C.: American Psychiatric Press.

Seto, M.C., Lalumière, M.L., Kuban, M. (1999). The sexual preferences of incest offenders. *Journal of Abnormal Psychology* 108(2): 267-272.

Sgroi, S.M. (1982). *Handbook of Clinical Intervention in Child Sexual Abuse.* Lexington, Massachusetts: Lexington Books.

Sheinberg, M. (1992). Navigating treatment bypasses in the disclosure of incest: Combining ideas from feminism and social constructionism. *Family Process* 31: 201-216.

Shepher, J. (1983). *Incest: A Biosocial View.* New York: Academic Press.

Simari, C., Baskin, D. (1982). Incestuous experiences within homosexual populations: A preliminary study. *Archives of Sexual Behavior* 11: 329-344.

Sirles, E.A., Franke, P.J. (1989). Factors influencing mothers' reactions to intrafamily sexual abuse. *Child Abuse & Neglect* 13: 131-139.

Smith, H., Israel, E. (1987). Sibling incest: A study of the dynamics of 25 cases. *Child Abuse & Neglect* 11: 101-108.

State v. Warner, 291 P. 307 (1932).

Streicher-Bremer, J.L. (2001). Expanding the understanding of heroin addiction in women who were sexually abused as children. *Dissertation Abstracts International, Section B: The Sciences and Engineering*, vol. 61, II-B 6150.

Summit, R. (1983). The child sexual abuse accommodation syndrome. *Child Abuse & Neglect* 7: 177-193.

Taubman, S. (1984). Incest in context. *Social Work* 29(1): 35-40.

Thornhill, N.W. (1991). An evolutionary analysis of rules regulating human inbreeding and marriage. *Behavioral and Brain Sciences* 14: 247-293.

Tolkinnen, K. (2003). Expert says Alabama is lagging in raising its marriage age. *Mobile Register,* March 30.

Trickett, P.K., Putnam, F.W. (1993). The impact of child sexual abuse on females: Toward a developmental, psychobiological integration. *Psychological Science* 4: 81-87.

Turell, S.C., Armsworth, M.W. (2000). Differentiating incest survivors who self-mutilate. *Child Abuse & Neglect* 24(2): 237-249.

United Nations Children's Fund. (2001). Early marriage, child spouses. Innocenti Digest 7, March. Available at http://www.unicef-icdc. org/publications/pdf/digest7e.pdf. Last accessed May 24, 2004.

United Nations Office for Drug Control and Crime Prevention. (2000). The Protocol to Prevent, Suppress, and Punish Trafficking in Persons, Especially Women and Children. Available at http://odccp.org// trafficking_protocol.html. Last accessed February, 2002.

Utah Code Annotated § 76-7-102 (2004).

Van den Berghe, P.L. (1983). Human inbreeding avoidance: Culture in nature. *The Behavioral and Brain Sciences* 6: 91-123.

Van der Kolk, B. (1994). The body keeps the score: Memory and the evolving psychobiology of posttraumatic stress. *Harvard Review of Psychiatry* January/February: 253-265.

Warner, E. (2004). Behind the wedding veil: Child marriage as a form of trafficking in girls. *American University Journal of Gender, Society, Policy & Law* 12: 233-271.

Weinberg, S.K. (1955). *Incest Behavior*. New York: Citadel.

Westerlund, E. (1983). Counseling women with histories of incest. *Women and Therapy* 2: 17-31.

Westermark, E.A. (1891). *The History of Human Marriage*. London: Macmillan.

Williams, L.M. (1994). Recall of childhood trauma: A Prospective study of women's memories of child sexual abuse. *Journal of Consulting and Clinical Psychology* 62: 1167-1176.

Williams, L.M., Finkelhor, D. (1995). Paternal caregiving and incest: Test of a biosocial model. *American Journal of Orthopsychiatry* 65: 101-113.

Winnicott, D.W. (1958). The capacity to be alone. In *The Maturational Processes and the Facilitating Environment*. New York: International Universities Press, 1965.

Winnicott, D.W. (1952). Psychoses and child care. In *Collected Papers: Through Paediatrics to Psycho-Analysis*. London, Tavistock, 1958.

CHAPTER 4

Commercial "Partnering": Sex Work, Trafficking, and Pornography

Introduction

This chapter focuses on health issues arising in the context of commercial partnering. Such partnering may be voluntary, as in the case of a sex worker who out of choice engages in sexual activity for profit, or involuntary, as in the case of a child sold into labor who is beaten into submission and forced to provide sexual favors to adult clientele. In circumstances involving involuntary sexual activity, "partnering" becomes a misnomer. The commercial exchange for sex may be legal, as in the brothels of Nevada or the Netherlands, or illegal, such as that which occurs outside the parameters of legalized commercial sex, such as that in illegal brothels, bars, nightclubs, massage parlors, bathhouses, private dwellings, and public spaces. It may take the form of direct solicitation and exchange, such as that which occurs when a sex worker receives payment from his or her client, or indirectly, as in the case of a porn star who engages in sex with another individual but is paid by a third party, or a sex worker who is matched to a client by a pimp and is paid only a fraction of the client's remuneration by the pimp. The commercial enterprise may be small, or may involve a large and complex network of multiple middlemen. Just as the circumstances and settings of commercial sexual activity differ so greatly, so too do some of the health issues that attend commercial partnering.

Sex Work

The term *prostitution* has been defined as "the act or instance of offering or devoting one's talent to an unworthy use or cause (*American Heritage Dictionary*) or "the performance of a sexual act for material gain" (Andesron and Estes, 1998: 152). It has often been used to denote sex work engaged in for monetary remuneration. This usage fails to acknowledge those instances of exchange involving the receipt of gifts by a woman from a married man not her husband, in appreciation of her continuing companionship and sexual favors; the partnering of a man and a woman following a first date during which he pays for dinner and drinks; or the receipt by a woman or a man of gifts within the context of a loveless, cold marriage. However, if the woman

requests money, specifically in exchange for sex, if she solicits and accepts payment in some form for sex, then she is a prostitute. The request for payment, not the sexual act and not receiving something of value for sexual services, is the action being proscribed. The name of the crime in many venues, in fact, recognizes this communication basis: soliciting. In each case, the same behaviors may occur with respect to sex, the same outcomes may occur with respect to sex, and the same payments are made. The only difference occurs in the communication of a request from the woman or an offer from the man, and this makes the instance prostitution. If this is true, then prostitution is clearly a crime of speech and communication, not a crime of sexual behavior or payment for sexual favors (Steinfatt, 2002: 14).

Additionally, the use of the term implies that money has been exchanged for something without value. If this were, indeed, the case, it would be unlikely that so many individuals would part with their money for something having no value.

However, the application of the term has actually varied across time, place, and culture (Bullough and Bullough, 1964). As an example, in Romania during the rule of Ceaucescu, which spanned

23 years from his assumption of the presidency in 1965 to his violent overthrow in 1989, single women found in hotel rooms with men were routinely charged with the crime of prostitution, although the male could be a boyfriend or lover (Harsanyi, 1993). Currently, law enforcement would not consider a single woman and a man sharing a hotel room to signify prostitution, absent additional indications of such. In the United States, prostitution as an activity has at varying times been designated as illegal but tolerated, behavior; illegal behavior that was to be eradicated; or legal behavior if confined to specified zones (Rosen, 1982).

Attitudes towards prostitution have also varied. As one researcher observed, "What is deviant during one period of history may receive public toleration in another, and prostitution appears to be particularly susceptible to cycles of public toleration and persecution" (Rosen, 1982: 39). In the minds of onlookers, prostitution has variously been associated and/or equated with feeblemindedness; broken homes; disease; lower social status; sterility caused by venereal disease; immigrant women; race suicide; sexual overdevelopment; a lack of morality; the victimization and corruption of unwilling, innocent young girls; an economic response to poverty; the political subordination of women; and an example of male exploitation and coercion of women (Rosen, 1982). And, although the image of sex work has most often involved sexual favors being delivered by women to men, it is clear that male sex work exists in the United States (Morse, Simon, & Burchfiel, 1999) and elsewhere (Aggleton, 1999; Steinfatt, 2002).

Increasingly, the relationship between the sex worker and the paying customer has become more complex with the appearance of middlemen and the development of prostitution into a major commercialized enterprise. Although varying by time and place, this enterprise may involve a widespread network consisting of police, politicians, bartenders, waiters, chauffeurs, cabdrivers, madams, pimps, landlords, real estate agents, business owners, and others (Rosen, 1982).

Women engaged in sex work have been variously portrayed as victimized and unknowing or morally depraved. However, the motivations for entering sex work appear significantly more complex. Many women may have been abused as either children or adult partners and began sex work as a means of survival. Some women may be forced into it by their male partners. Still others choose sex work as a legitimate means of earning a living (Stetson, 2004). One study of prostitution in the United States during the early twentieth century reported that the poverty that motivated women to engage in sex work in the brothels often resulted from the death of or abandonment by the woman's husband, low wages due to seasonal employment of the woman and/or her husband or partner, the husband's loss of employment, or the abandonment of the woman by her sexual partner following an early love affair and the discovery that she was pregnant (Rosen 1982). Working class women were often barred from social and economic competition because of their social class and gender; commercial sex work provided a means to move forward economically. Some middle-class women engaged in prostitution were abandoned by their families when they became pregnant; prostitution provided a means of support for themselves and their child. Still other single middle-class women engaged in prostitution after they were ostracized as moral deviants for their sexual behavior, which would have been acceptable but for the fact that they were women. Still others used prostitution as a means of rebellion against their families and society (Rosen, 1982). O'Neill (1999) has reported similar pathways to commercial prostitution among sex workers in more recent times: a need to reduce an increased debt burden, peer pressure, pressure from pimp boyfriends, homelessness and a need to earn a living, a desire for financial independence and, unlike past eras, a need for money for substance use.

Albert (2001) reported from her ethnographic study of commercial sex workers in a legalized Nevada brothel that multiple motivations existed for women's entry into the profession. Some had entered to make more money; the women averaged six customers per day and received payment between $300 and $1500 per day, depending upon the services requested. Others related that they enjoyed sex. Still others engaged in commercial sex work on a temporary basis, to cover unpaid bills or because their husbands told them they needed more money. Others noted that their customers were often obsessed with specific body parts, such as breasts, buttocks, or blond hair; many of the women felt that their services served a healing purpose. Many of the women also shared a situation characterized by financial hardship and an edict from their pimp boyfriend or husband to contribute more financially.

Less than half of the women in Albert's study reported having been sexually abused as children. Many of the women came from intact two-parent families. Two-thirds of the women were observant in one of the major faiths (usually Catholicism, Protestantism, and Judaism). Less than one-half sold sex outside of the brothels and fewer than 10% had been street-based sex workers before coming to the brothel. Most of the women reported that they had satisfying sexual relations outside of work, but that they had to do something different than what they did at work in order to become aroused.

Stereotypes abound regarding male sex workers, alternately portraying them as heterosexual hustlers or teenage runaway prostitutes (Davies and Simpson, 1990). Research indicates that the demographic characteristics of male sex workers vary depending upon time and place. In the U.S., male sex workers are often between the ages of 18 and 40, are relatively well-educated, are of diverse ethnic and racial groups, and various sexual orientations (Morse, Simon, and Burchfield, 1999). Many of them may have left their homes at an early age and/or were subject to physical and sexual abuse (Caulkins and Coombs, 1976; Morse, Simon, Osofsky, Balson, and Gaumier, 1991). Studies of male sex workers in various locales within the U.K. indicate that they may have a regular boy- or girlfriend and/or casual sexual partners of either sex (Davies and Feldman, 1999). Distinctions are often made between regular and casual customers; relationships with regular customers may involve caring as well as a financial transaction (Davies and Feldman, 1999).

A study of child and adolescent prostitution in Los Angeles, California found that the young commercial sex workers often fell into one of several categories: those providing call services individually or through agencies; female street-based workers who worked for themselves; female street-based workers who worked for pimps; amateur sex workers who hustled part-time for themselves or their boyfriends; boy street hustlers; weekender hustlers, who engaged in sex work for the excitement or for party money; professional hustlers aged 19 to 22, who worked for a few years in the sex industry and who may also have participated in the porn industry; survivors under the age of 18, who had been pushed out of their homes and often lacked education, work skills, and skills necessary for independent living; and survivors under the age of 14, who were often runaways (Nicholsen, 1981). Many of these children had poor relationships with adults, had suffered sexual abuse as children, and were at risk of violence on the streets.

Not all brothels were or are alike. Rather, they cater to different clientele, willing to pay more or less for the services that they are to receive (Albert, 2001; Rosen, 1982). Working conditions for the women employed in brothels also vary and are often dependent upon the practices of the brothel owner or manager (Albert, 2001). While some managers appear to be respectful of the women who work in their brothels, other managers may go so far as to require the women to disrobe and submit to their examination of their bodies to ascertain the quality of their physique and to check for track marks. In some Nevada brothels, women may keep personal supplies of condoms and lubricants, while in others, the owner confiscates these supplies and demands that the women repurchase everything from the brothel at inflated prices, much like miners being forced to purchase their goods from the company store. In Nevada, HIV testing is required as a condition of legal employment as a sex worker; once employed, the workers are required to have tests on a monthly basis for HIV and syphilis and on a weekly basis for gonorrhea and Chlamydia (Albert, 2001). Such stringent health requirements clearly do not prevail across all existing brothels, regardless of their location (Zimmerman, Yun, Schvab et al., 2003).

Relatively little research has been conducted relating to the individuals who purchase sexual favors. It has been argued that the client of a prostitute or sex worker does not want only an orgasm, because there are other means of achieving orgasm. It has further been argued that he does not want sex, because sex can be obtained from willing partners who do not wish to be paid. One man explained his underlying motivation for utilizing the services of a sex worker:

Of all the commentators, *Screw* publisher Al Goldstein was the most honest, reporting a story about the night he spent $100 on an escort. "It was splendid, rollicking sex. When it was over, I felt like willing my body to science. And then she left. She left. As the supreme final act in our opera of fucking, her leaving was like a cherry on a sundae, a sumptuous dessert after a seven-course meal, a plunge into cool water after running a marathon. That's when I had my glistening realization. I realized I wasn't paying this woman for sex. I was paying her for the luxury of her leaving after sex (Peterson, 1995: 52).

Trafficking

Definitions and Conceptual Frameworks

Trafficking has been defined in a number of ways through various protocols and conventions, as indicated in Table 3, below. As can be seen from these definitions, the concept of trafficking in women and children for the purpose of sexual exploitation has often overlapped with definitions and perceptions of prostitution. Indeed, officials in some countries dispute the existence of trafficking resulting in involuntary commercial sex work, believing that women who are trafficked across international borders and ultimately engage in sex work do so of their own volition, without deception or coercion and, therefore, despite having been trafficked, do not need and/or deserve protection (Altink, 1995). This debate essentially hinges on the question of the role of consent and whether a distinction should be made between voluntary and forced prostitution. As seen below, the definition of trafficking that has been adopted in the United Nations Protocol eliminates the focus on consent in order to emphasize punishment of traffickers, regardless of whether the woman consented to prostitution. This approach fails to acknowledge that some individuals may choose to be trafficked to engage in commercial sex work, and it may be the conditions under which they work that result in brutalization. Accordingly, this approach has been criticized for its underlying assumption that no one would choose to be trafficked or to engage in prostitution (Bruch, 2004).

The concept of trafficking similarly overlaps with that of illegal migration. Some individuals may actively enlist the aid of traffickers to cross into another country. The individuals may be motivated by any number of reasons, such as a search for economic opportunities, flight from persecution and/or torture, or to join family members who migrated previously. Regardless of their motive, the trafficked individuals may be caught up in a small- or large-scale enterprise that focuses on the trafficking of human beings as commodities. The relationship between prostitution, trafficking, and immigration is illustrated by Figure 3, below.

As illustrated by this figure, the intersection of trafficking, sex work, and immigration may encompass any of the following situations, among others:

Table 3. Definitions of Trafficking

Use of Definition	Definition of Trafficking
Archivantikul et al., 1998	a child who is recruited and transported from one place to another across a national border, legally or illegally, with or without the child's consent, usually but not always organized by an intermediary: parents, family member, teacher, procurer, or local authority. At the destination, the child is coerced or semi-forced (by deceptive information) to engage in activities under exploitative and abusive conditions
Bangladesh National Women Lawyers Association	All acts involved in the recruitment and/or transport of a woman (or child) within and across national borders for work or services (or marriage) by means of violence or threat of violence, abuse of authority or dominant position, debt bondage, deception or other forms of coercion (Ali, 1998)
Consultation Workshop of the Resistance Network, Bangladesh, 1999	Trafficking in women consists of all acts involved in the procurement, transportation, forced movement, and/or selling and buying of women within and/or across borders by fraudulent means, deception, coercion, direct and/or indirect threats, abuse of authority, for the purpose of placing a woman against her will without her consent in exploitative and abusive situations such as forced prostitution, forced marriage, bonded and forced labour, begging, organ trade, etc.

Continued

Table 3. (*Continued*)

Use of Definition	Definition of Trafficking
	Trafficking in children consists of all acts involved in the procurement, transportation, forced movement, and/or selling and buying of children within and/or across borders by fraudulent means, deception, coercion, direct and/or indirect threats, abuse of authority, for the purpose of placing a child against his or her will without consent in exploitative and abusive situations, such as commercial sexual abuse, forced marriage, bonded and forced labour, begging, camel jockeying and other sports, organ trade, etc.
Global Alliance against Trafficking in Women	All acts involved in the recruitment and/or transportation of a woman within and across national borders for work or services by means of violence or threat of violence, abuse of authority or dominant position, debt-bondage, deception or other forms of coercion (Archivantikul, 1998)
International Office of Migration (1999)	Trafficking occurs when a migrant is illicitly recruited and/or moved for the purpose of economically or otherwise exploiting the migrant, under conditions that violate their fundamental human rights.
United Nations' Protocol to Prevent, Suppress, and Punish Trafficking in Persons, Especially	the recruitment, transportation, transfer, harbouring or receipt of persons, by means of the threat or use of force or other forms of

Table 3. (*Continued*)

Use of Definition	Definition of Trafficking
Women and Children	coercion, of abduction, of fraud, of deception, of the abuse of power or of a position of vulnerability . . . or of the giving or receiving of payments or benefits to achieve the consent of a person having control over another person, for the purpose of exploitation. Exploitation shall include, at a minimum, the exploitation of the prostitution of others or other forms of sexual exploitation . . . forced labour or services, slavery or practices similar to slavery, servitude, or the removal of organs (United Nations Office for Drug Control and Crime Prevention, 2000).
U.S. Agency for International Development	The recruitment of girls/women by means of violence or threat, debt bondage, deception or coercion to act as sex workers under menace of penalty and for which the individual has not offered themselves voluntarily (Gazi et al., 2001, quoting Matt Friedman)
U.S. President's Interagency Council on Women	All acts involved in the recruitment, transport, harboring or sale of persons within national or across international borders through deception or fraud, coercion or force, or debt bondage for purposes of placing persons in situations of forced labor or services, such as forced prostitution or sexual services, domestic servitude, or other forms of slavery-like practices

- Legal immigration to a country, followed by voluntary trafficking within that country to engage in voluntary sex work under agreed upon conditions
- Legal immigration to a country followed by voluntary trafficking within that country to engage in voluntary sex work under forced conditions
- Legal immigration to a country, followed by involuntary trafficking within that country and forced sex work and sex work conditions
- Legal immigration to a country, followed by involuntary trafficking within that country and voluntary sex work but under forced conditions
- Illegal immigration to a country through voluntary trafficking for the purpose of engaging in voluntary sex work under agreed upon conditions
- Illegal immigration to a country through voluntary trafficking for the purpose of engaging in voluntary sex work, but under involuntary conditions

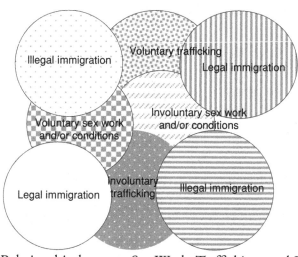

Figure 3. Relationship between Sex Work, Trafficking, and Immigration

- Illegal immigration to a country through voluntary trafficking, but forced to engage in involuntary sex work under unwanted work conditions
- Illegal immigration to a country through involuntary trafficking and forced to engage in involuntary sex work under forced conditions

Trafficking does not always result in involuntary sex work; individuals may be drafted into involuntary servitude in factories, domestic situations, sweat shops, and other commercial enterprises. Because the circumstances and perceptions of trafficking are so varied, as with other terms explored in this text, we lack a common language that encompasses all dimensions of the concept.

Governments and agencies have adopted varying approaches to trafficking. These have been classified into six distinct perspectives (Foundation of Women's Forum, citing Marjan Wijers, Foundation Against Trafficking in Women.), based upon their views towards trafficking, immigration, and sex work.

(1) The moral approach views trafficking as an evil that must be controlled. This approach focuses on the punishment of all parties involved, which may result in the stigmatization and punishment of the victims, as well as the perpetrators.

(2) The criminal approach seeks to improve international police cooperation and increase the effectiveness of prosecutions. This approach subordinates the interests of the trafficked women and children to the interests of the prosecution, and may result in the prosecution of the women for prostitution and/or illegal entry into the country (Foundation of Women's Forum, citing Marjan Wijers, Foundation Against Trafficking in Women). One commentator has explained:

Many governments take an approach of criminalizing all aspects of prostitution. Others criminalize only certain aspects or legalize and regulate other aspects. Because of the differing approaches, there has been debate over how, and whether, prostitution should be included within a definition of trafficking. Because it is both criminalized and stigmatized in many societies, this treatment reflects a judgment about prostitutes and prostitution, particularly when the prostitution is voluntary . . . The law enforcement approach struggles to reconcile two apparently conflicting views of prostitutes and prostitution—one that seeks to protect individuals from being trafficked into prostitution and another that seeks to exclude from protection those who willingly engage in the criminal conduct of prostitution, even if they have been trafficked to another country . . . . (Bruch, 2004: 18-19).

(3) The immigration perspective seeks stricter control of national boundaries and may also seek to regulate marriage between citizens and foreigners. The interests of the state are paramount. Individuals who are voluntarily trafficked may be identified as illegal immigrants and dealt with as illegal entrants pursuant to a country's immigration laws.

As an example, although U.S. immigration law offers some potential recourse for individuals who have been involuntarily trafficked and forced into sex work, the interests of the government in controlling the illegal activity are clearly paramount. A maximum of 5,000 "T" visas are available each year to individuals who are or who have been the victim of a severe form of trafficking in persons; are physically present in the United States or various territories, are under the age of 15 or have complied with any reasonable request for assistance in the investigation or prosecution of trafficking, and would suffer extreme hardship involving unusual or severe harm upon removal from the United States (Victims of Trafficking and Violence Protection Act, 2000). "Sex trafficking" is defined as "the recruitment, harboring, transportation, provision, or obtaining of a person for the purpose of a commercial sex act." "Severe trafficking" is defined by the law as

sex trafficking in which a commercial sex act is induced by force, fraud, or coercion, or in which the person induced to perform such act has not attained 18 years of age; or

the recruitment, harboring, transportation, provision, or obtaining of a person for labor or services, through the use of force, fraud, or coercion for the purpose of subjection to involuntary servitude, peonage, debt bondage, or slavery (Victims of Trafficking and Violence Protection Act, 2000).

This visa allows the individual to remain in the United States only for a temporary period of time. Additionally, even though the issuance of the visa is based on the individual's cooperation in the investigation or prosecution of the trafficking, witness protection is not generally provided to the trafficked individual.

Alternatively, a "U" visa, which also allows an individual to remain in the United States only temporarily, is potentially available to up to 10,000 persons each year who have suffered substantial physical or mental abuse as a result of having been the victim of trafficking or various other enumerated offenses; possesses information about the crime; and is, has been, or is likely to be helpful to law enforcement authorities in the investigation or prosecution of the crime, which must have been in violation of U.S. law or committed in the U.S. or a designated territory or possession (Victims of Trafficking and Violence Protection Act, 2000). Again, witness protection is generally unavailable.

(4) The human rights perspective sees prostitution itself as a violation of human rights that should be abolished or, alternatively, views the conditions under which women engage in commercial sex work (deceit, abuse, violence, etc.) as violative of human rights.

(5) The public order approach views trafficking as a problem of public order and/or public health and focuses on control, such as that effectuated through medical examinations, as a solution.

(6) The labor perspective holds that trafficking in women is the result of women's relatively low social and economic status and advocates the establishment of increased economic rights and opportunities for women as a solution (Foundation of Women's Forum, 1998, citing Marjan Wijers, Foundation Against Trafficking in Women).

Patterns of Trafficking

Trafficking occurs both within a country and across international borders. The International Organisation for Migration (2001) has estimated that between 700,000 and two million women and children are trafficked across international borders each year, but the estimates have been as high as four million per year (Gushulak & MacPherson, 2000). Accurate numbers are difficult to calculate due to varying and disputed definitions of trafficking, the criminal nature of the activity, and the lack of attention that it receives in many countries.

In Asia, major source countries include Thailand, the Philippines, Myanmar, Vietnam, Cambodia, Bangladesh, and Nepal; transit and destination countries there include Thailand, Malaysia, Japan, India, and Pakistan. The majority of women and children trafficked in the region are to be forced into the sex industry. The majority of children forced into the sex industry in Sri Lanka are boys (O'Neill, 1999). However, some are also trafficked for marriages purposes due to the weighty expense of dowries, for commercial sexual services that are linked to religious practices (India and Nepal), and for other forms of bonded labor, such as begging (O'Neill, 1999; Wennerholm, 2002).

Many trafficked women originate from former Communist-regime countries (Russia, Romania, Albania, Kosovo, the Baltic States, the Czech Republic, Poland) and former Central Asian republics of the Soviet Union (Kazakhstan, Kyrgyszstan, Tajikstan). Other countries of origin include various countries in Latin America (Cuba, the Dominican Republic, Mexico, Argentina, Brazil, Colombia, Peru, Paraguay, and Uruguay) and in Africa (Ghana, Nigeria, Ethiopia, and Mali). Women in Central and West Africa may be trafficked for the purpose of domestic labor and children to perform work as domestics, as plantation laborers, or as sex workers.

The United States appears to be a major destination country for trafficked persons from almost all regions, with the possible exception of Africa. Canada is both a major destination country and a transit country for further trafficking to the United States (McDonald, Moore, & Timoshkina, 2000). Western European countries serve as receiving countries for trafficked persons from Latin America and Eastern Europe. Trafficked persons from these regions are often destined for the United States, Japan, and countries in Western Europe (Wennerholm, 2002), while those from the Central Asian republics are often smuggled into countries of the Middle East, as well as Turkey, Greece, and the Ukraine (International Organisation for Migration, 2001). Destination countries for persons trafficked from Africa include Nigeria, Côte d'Ivoire, Lebanon, Libya, Kuwait, Saudi Arabia, the U.S, and Western European nations (International Organisation for Migration, 2001). Israel has also served as a destination country for trafficked persons from several Eastern European and Latin American countries (Wennerholm, 2002).

Although it would appear from media coverage that trafficking in human beings for commercial use as sex slaves in the United States is a relatively recent phenomenon, such activity is one of longstanding. During the mid- to late-1800s in the United States, the emphasis on the victimization of women in sex work led a number of reformers to focus on the issue of "white slavery," which referred to instances in which women were forcibly recruited into prostitution or were prevented from leaving it (Rosen, 1982). Foreign women brought to the United States were declared by those meeting them to be the wives or relatives of the men, who were actually procurers. The women were enticed to the U.S. with promises of marriage and/or employment; their families often received a payment. The women were then sold to houses of prostitution, where they were "broken in" by being drugged, raped and beaten, and then were imprisoned in cells with little light or air, known as "cribs." They were rarely allowed to leave and, after some time, few attempted to leave due to internalized shame, disgrace, self-blame, and a loss of faith in human nature. Of the procurers convicted under the Mann Act (see below) during this same period of time, 72.5% were U.S.-born (Rosen, 1982).

Although trafficking in women and children is not a recent phenomenon, data indicate that there may be a recent upsurge in such activity. Table 4, below, lists the various factors that are believed to contribute to this upsurge, although the relative importance of each factor varies depending upon the specific country and time period.

Stages and Modes of Trafficking

Five stages of trafficking have been identified: the pre-departure stage; the travel and transit stage; the destination stage; the detention, deportation, and criminal evidence stage; and the integration and reintegration stage (Zimmerman, Yun, Schvab et al., 2003). The demarcation of these periods is indicated in Table 5, below.

Several methods of trafficking have been identified, that fall along a spectrum of lesser or greater severity of abuse. Individuals may experience situations at one or more points along this spectrum, depending upon their individual circumstances. Points along this continuum, from the most abusive to the least abusive, are as follows:

- Victims are forced and/or kidnapped and trafficked.
- Victims are given false information and trafficked into other types of activities than were originally promised.
- Victims realize the nature of the work, such as sex work, but are unaware of the conditions under which they will be working.
- Victims are aware of both the nature of the work that they will be doing and the conditions under which they will be working but are not aware or are not able to foresee the level of difficulty associated with the situations that they will encounter.
- Laborers realize the nature of the work and the working conditions they will face, but are not given any alternatives.
- Laborers realize the nature of the work and the work conditions and are able to select alternatives.

This last scenario is illustrated by the decision of some women to engage in sex work in response to difficult or abusive circumstances,

Table 4. Factors Influencing the Incidence of Trafficking in Women and Children for Sexual Exploitation

Factor	Examples
Historical context	Formation of cross-border families due to political divisions between nations, e.g. U.S-Mexico, Pakistan-India, and frequent cross-border traffic for commercial reasons (Gazi, 2001)
Geographical context	Natural disasters such as flooding or drought, leading to increased poverty, separation of families and search for employment; (Gazi et al., 2001)
Socioeconomic context	High prevalence of poverty leading to search for employment outside of country, sale of children by families; high prevalence of female-headed households; low levels of education limiting economic opportunities (Gazi et al., 2001); difficulty accessing the formal labor market in country of immigration (International Organization for Migration, 2003)
Cultural context	Cultural norms promoting early and arranged marriage of girls; vulnerability of women to abuse/sale by relatives due to dissatisfaction with bridal dowry (cf. Nagi, 1993); stigma and ostracism of women who have been deserted or divorced by their husbands; mores dictating female dependency on men; desire of migrant men abroad for sex workers with common cultural and linguistic background (Gazi et al., 2001); sexual harassment and demanded sexual favors in the workplace making payment for sex a desirable alternative (Foundation of Women's Forum, 1998)

Continued

Table 4. (*Continued*)

Factor	Examples
Political context	Collapse of the Soviet Union with resulting economic hardships and dislocation (Cwikel et al., 2004; Foundation of Women's Forum, 1998); corruption of law enforcement personnel, facilitating trafficking; lack of shelter and support for women in distress (Gazi et al., 2001); illegality of prostitution and probable prosecution and/or deportation of trafficking victims for legal and/or immigration violations (International Organization for Migration, 2003)

Table 5. Stages of Trafficking

Stage of Trafficking	Definition	Characteristics of Stage
Pre-departure stage	"The period before a woman enters the trafficking situation"	May be characterized by poverty, difficult or disrupted relationships
Travel and transit stage	Commences at the time of recruitment when a woman is forced to depart or agrees to depart with a trafficker, regardless of whether or not she knows that she is being trafficked, and extends until she arrives at her work destination, regardless of the number of transit points between the point of origin and the point of work	Possibly dangerous modes of transportation, evasion of discovery

Table 5. (*Continued*)

Stage of Trafficking	Definition	Characteristics of Stage
Destination stage	Begins when the woman is at the location where she is put to work and is the target of coercion, violence, exploitation, debt-bondage or other forms of abuse associated with trafficking	May be subject to physical and sexual violence as a means of control; deprivation of food, human contact, valued items; held in solitary confinement; forced to use drugs or alcohol; deprived of earnings
Detention, deportation, and criminal evidence stage	Refers to the period of time during which the woman is in the custody of law enforcement or immigration authorities for alleged violation of criminal or immigration laws or is voluntarily or involuntarily cooperating with authorities in legal proceedings against individuals perpetrating the trafficking or abuse	Women rarely provided with health assistance by authorities; conditions often inadequate
Integration and re-integration stage	A long-term and multi-faceted process that concludes when the woman achieves active membership in the	

Continued

Table 5. (*Continued*)

Stage of Trafficking	Definition	Characteristics of Stage
	economic, cultural, civil, and political life of a country and "perceives that she has oriented and is accepted"	

Based on Zimmerman, Yun, Schvab et al., 2003.

such as widowhood, desertion by a husband, or sexual abuse. The woman realizes the nature of the work and the work conditions and is able to choose how she will engage in sex work. However, it is possible that she will later be forcefully or deceptively trafficked and forced to perform sexual services (Archavanitkul, 1998; Gazi et al., 2001; Khan and Arefeen, 1988). A study based on interviews with 55 trafficked sex workers in Israel found that all but 2 of them knew before leaving their country of origin that they would be engaging in sex work (Chudakov, Ilan, Belmaker, and Cwikel, 2002). However, 17% were sold to a brothel owner against their wishes and 64% were transferred to other places of work without their consent. Eighteen percent of the women were neither transferred nor sold; all of these women had obtained legal resident status in Israel (Cwikel, Ilan, and Chudakov, 2003), suggesting that legal status may be a critical factor in the trafficking dynamic and the fate of trafficked women.

Often, a woman is tricked or coerced by the trafficker or an intermediary. The procurement process may involve kidnapping or abduction, promises of a better job, a promise of marriage or a forced marriage, the sale of young girls by their parents or guardians, the sale of women by their husbands, the deception of girls and women for legal or illegal immigration, and/or the rape or abuse of women and girls (Gazi et al., 2001). An employee of the U.S. Agency for International Development characterized the procurement process as a

breach in trust. Trafficking takes place, because an individual who has trust with either an individual girl, or family makes false promises of a better future to another individual and that is believable and offers them to say, I, as an individual, may decide to go or may allow a family member to go. It really comes down to that misconception whether it is trafficking or migration. A trafficker lies, provokes, offers promises, offers opportunities, and says here is a better future for you. Not a year from now but immediately your future will suddenly get better. This is what trafficking is all about" (Gazi et al., 2001: 16, quoting Matt Friedman).

Several studies that examined modes of trafficking have documented the role played by trusted individuals and family members in enticing young girls and women with promises of a better future (International Organization for Migration, 2003; Rajbhandari and Rajbhandari, 1997; Women's Publishing House and Media Resource Organization, 1998). When questioned about their trafficking activities, intermediaries and traffickers interviewed in prison enumerated their strategies for identifying a potential trafficking victim: a woman in search of a job or a love affair, who could be tempted by false promises of marriage or a false marriage (Gazi et al., 2001; International Organization for Migration, 1996). Such individuals could be found at bus stations and border crossings, while others might already be employed as sex workers. Uneducated individuals arriving at these points from rural areas appear to be particularly vulnerable to such strategies. Traffickers may "take orders" from their clients and search for women with specified characteristics and then transport them to their clients' homes; this practice has been documented, for instance, in northern Norway (Foundation of Women's Forum, 1998).

Media accounts and reports from international organizations have documented the circumstances under which women, young girls, and young males have been forced to engage in sex work and the conditions under which they must service their customers. In the United States, newspapers reported, for instance, the 1996 confinement of Russian women to a massage parlor in Bethesda, Maryland, following their response to a job ad for work in the United States, and the 1998 arrest of the Cadena family for their operation of a brothel in North Carolina, South Carolina, and Florida using the forced services of girls from Mexico (Stetson, 2004). Many times, the involuntary sex workers are confined against their will in unsanitary and brutal environments, with no ability to contact anyone who might be of assistance. Failed attempts to transmit messages through seemingly sympathetic customers may result in further brutalization as punishment. Condoms may or may not be supplied and, clearly, in these circumstances, the trafficked person has no ability to obtain them independently (Zimmerman, Yun, Schvab et al., 2003). Such circumstances are a far cry from the conditions that prevail at some of Nevada's legalized brothels in which women voluntarily engage in sex work and, not surprisingly, carry with them different and/or greater health risks.

The Legal Context

Trafficking in human beings is in violation of both international and U.S. law. The United Nations' Protocol to Prevent, Suppress, and Punish Trafficking in Persons, Especially Women and Children obligates signatories to "take all necessary measures to repeal or abolish any law, regulation or administrative provisions by virtue of which persons who are engaged in, or are suspected of engaging in, prostitution are subject to either special registration or to the possession of a special document or to any exceptional requirements for supervision or notification."

In the United States, the Mann Act, formally titled the "White Slave Traffic Act" was enacted in 1910, making it a federal felony to

transport or cause to be transported or aid or assist in obtaining transportation for, or in transporting, in interstate or foreign commerce, or in any Territory or in the District of Columbia, any woman or girl for the purpose of prostitution or debauchery, or for any other immoral purpose to induce, entice, or compel such woman or girl to become a prostitute or give herself up to debauchery, or to engage in any other immoral practice (quoted in Stetson, 2004: 246).

The language of the Mann Act has since been amended and currently provides for the prosecution of individuals engaged in the transportation of an individual through interstate or foreign commerce with the intent that the individual engage in prostitution. Conviction carries a penalty of no more than five years imprisonment or a fine, but not both (18 U.S.C. section 1952, 2005).

Enforcement of country-specific and/or international laws prohibiting trafficking is rendered more difficult in those jurisdictions that provide for legal sex work. As an example, sex work is a legal form of employment in Austria that requires registration with the designated authorities and periodic health examinations; proceeds from such employment are taxable. Non-Austrian sex workers may have entered the country legally as tourists and then engage in sex work without either a work permit or a residence permit. In some local jurisdictions, police issue the requisite permit to engage in sex work without verifying legal resident status, believing that a focus on registration is preferable and will prevent the sex industry from moving underground and out of control. Illegally engaging in sex work subjects a woman to likely deportation for illegally crossing into the country, illegally residing in the country, and/or illegally working. As a consequence, women who are trafficked and in need of assistance are discouraged from seeking help from law enforcement authorities if they have been trafficked and forced to perform sex work. Additionally, their illegal status and consequent isolation serves to increase their dependence on their traffickers. Identification of the traffickers is also difficult because the women often know only the individuals who served as intermediaries for the traffickers (International Organization for Migration, 1996). A similar situation has been reported in Turkey (International Organization for Migration, 2003).

Pornography

Defining Pornography

Definitions of pornography clearly vary over time, culture, and place. The Concise Oxford Dictionary of Current English defines pornography as "the explicit description or exhibition of sexual activity in literature, films, etc. intended to stimulate erotic rather than aesthetic or emotional feelings" (Allen, 1990). In the United States, the legal classification of a writing, video, song, or other endeavor as pornography rests on a determination of whether an average person, applying contemporary community standards, would find that the work, taken as a whole, appeals to prurient interests; whether the work depicts in a patently offensive manner sexual conduct defined by closely drafted relevant state law; or whether the work, taken as a whole, lacks serious literary, artistic, political, or scientific value (*Miller v. California*, 1972). In contrast, annotations to the Criminal Code of Canada indicate that the courts have delineated three categories of pornography: explicit sex with violence, explicit sex that is without violence but subjects individuals to dehumanizing or degrading treatment, and explicit sex without violence that is neither dehumanizing nor degraing (Greenberg and Rosenberg, 2000). As in the United States, the ultimate determination of whether a communication or writing constitutes pornography is determined by reference to community standards of acceptability, which often turns on the degree of harm and degradation contained in the work.

A distinction is often made between pornography and erotica. Erotica has been defined as "sexually explicit material that depicts adult men and women consensually involved in pleasurable, nonviolent, nondegrading sexual interactions (Seto, Maric, and Barbaree, 2001: 37). In contrast, pornography involves depictions of sexual interactions in which one or more of the participants is objectified and rendered powerless or nonconsenting (Marshall and Barrett, 1990). Degrading pornography may portray people, usually women, as submissive or hypersexual individuals who derive pleasure from the sex act despite, or because of, the degradation and humiliation (Fisher and Barak, 1991). In its most extreme forms, pornography depicts acts of violence, torture, degradation, and mutilation of victims, who are most frequently females (MacKinnon, 1987). It has been argued that the goal of pornography is to produce sexual arousal in response to the sexual abuse of women (MacKinnon, 1987).

A significant body of research exists that addresses the relationship between pornography and the subsequent behavior and attitudes of its viewers (e.g., Dietz and Evans, 1982; Donnerstein and Berkowitz, 1981; Donnerstein and Linz, 1986; Linz, Donnerstein, and Penrod, 1984; Linz, Donnerstein, and Penrod, 1987; Zilmann and Bryant, 1982; Zillmann and Bryant, 1984). The discussion here focuses, instead, on the context in which pornography is produced and the health implications for those engaged in the "partnering" that comprises the pornographic product.

The Pornography Industry and Conditions of Employment

Relatively little empirical research has focused on the nature of the pornography industry and the working conditions and characteristics of those who are employed to perform the sex acts that are depicted in films, videos, and magazines. Much of the data that are available result from government investigations and inquiries.

It has been estimated that the production of more than three-quarters of all of the pornographic films and videos made in the United States occurs in and around the Los Angeles area (Attorney General's Commission on Pornography, 1986). Production costs are often kept to a minimum, and the same individual may serve as producer, director, and scriptwriter. The performers are often secured through an agent who specializes in recruiting individuals to perform in sexually explicit films.

The Attorney General's Commission on Pornography (1986) concluded that the distribution of pornographic videos and films appears to be controlled by one individual, with operations and controlled organizations throughout the United States. In addition, the Commission found that "significant portions of the pornographic magazine industry, the peep show industry, and the pornographic film industry are either directly operated or closely controlled by La Cosa Nostra members or very close associates."

Testimony provided to the Commission indicated that the vast majority of performers/models who appear in pornographic films and videos are relatively young. Many come from families characterized by divorce, the early death of a parent, and/or intense family conflict. Many have been sexually abused as children. Clearly, in the absence of systematic sampling and inquiry, it is impossible to determine the generalizability of these findings to all those who work as actors/models in the pornography industry.

Many of the women recruited into the work were originally recruited as nude models or adult models, and only later discovered that the work involved sexual activity. The agents who recruit them receive a daily fee for each model that they provide. Force may be used by filmmakers or by pimp boyfriends to "convince" the women to participate. One law enforcement officer testified to the

Commission:

Coercion comes in, especially like some of these witnesses have testified, in the area of anal sex, which many of the models don't want to get into. It really comes into a factor in the bondage and S&M type films. I have talked to models and I have seen films where it's quite obvious that the model has no idea as to what they were getting into. Part of an S&M film, when they start torturing the victim, tying them, whipping them and putting cigarettes out on their body, is the showing of pain. This is what sexually excites some people.

Obviously we are not dealing with people that can act, so they can't act the pain. Therefore the pain is very real. It's quite apparent these people do not realize what they have gotten into once they start the filming (Attorney General's Commission on Pornography, 1986).

Workdays are often 12 to 14 hours long; videos usually require three days and films require seven days to shoot. A video or film performer is expected to engage in at least two sex scenes in a production. Models may have anywhere from 24 to 32 different sexual partners in a month within the context of their work. In general, the actors/models do not have the option of using condoms or employing other safer sex strategies. In heterosexually-oriented pornography, women are expected to engage in scenes with women and/or men, while men engage in sex with only women. In pornography to be marketed to gay men, women do not appear at all.

The actors/models are paid by sex scene; at the time of the Commission's report, the standard rate was $200 to $250 per sex scene. Many of the women who participated in filming did so for economic reasons. One woman testified:

A lot of women are hurt or crazy women under stress. Yes, most women come in under a lot of stress. They're usually desperate when they first come in-maybe they need money for some emergency, like I did, or they've gone as long as they can doing odds and ends or working at (menial) jobs, and they finally just have to pay their bills. I met a woman whose kid was in the hospital, and I met lots of women who were financially strapped. There were also many illegal aliens who couldn't work regular jobs even if they had the skills because they didn't have their green cards . . . [T]hey certainly know how to get you to do what they want. Some women are so bad off that they just go immediately into hard-core films (Attorney General's Commission on Pornography, 1986).

It appears that one's career in the pornographic film industry is relatively short, and may span only a few months or years. Few women remain in the business after the age of 30, unless they are able to work their way into production or management positions; few men remain in the business for more than a year.

Commercial Partnering and Health

Reproductive Health

Gynecological problems are the most frequent health problem among trafficked women (Zimmerman, Yun, Schvab et al., 2003). Women who have been forced into sexual activity through trafficking have reported unintended pregnancies and the termination of those pregnancies in the country of destination. A number of the abortions resulted in complications (Zimmerman, Yun, Schvab et al., 2003).

Women have also reported undiagnosed and untreated pelvic pain. Of 55 women trafficked to Israel for sex work, 43% reported having had gynecologic problems during the previous five years (Cwikel, Ilan, and Chudakov, 2003). At the time of the interviews, 49% reported having current vaginal pain, 35% had pelvic pain, 31% experienced vaginal numbing, and an additional 27% had pelvic numbing.

Relationships

It appears that relatively little research has been conducted on the implications for relationships of voluntary or involuntary participation in commercial sex work. Albert's (2001) ethnography of women working in a Nevada brothel indicates that most of the women reported sexually satisfying relationships outside of work, but that they had to do something different than what they did at work in order to become aroused. Testimony presented to that Attorney General's Commission on Pornography in this regard often focused on the difficulties that such work posed to relationships. William Margold testified:

Whenever I'm interviewing someone who wants to get into porn, I always ask them, "Do you have anybody that you will hurt by doing this?" It would be ideal if someone had no relatives-disenfranchised human being devoid of any past that would haunt them and any kind of present or future that they could destroy. If it's a man, he also better be single because, unless he's married to the most magnanimous of women, it will tear her insides out.

One man, who had begun making adult films at the age of 17, stated, "I don't know, I feel scared to have a sexual relationship with a girl. I don't know what it's going to be like or if I am going to be too rough."

Safer Sex and Infectious Disease

The context in which sex work occurs and the meaning of the context to the women engaged in sex work may be closely related to the level of HIV risk. A study of sex workers in Belize, for instance, found that local women who offered services through bars did not define their exchanges for money as prostitution due to the stigma associated with that activity. Rather, they defined themselves as being in intimate relationships with their clients (Kane, 1998). They also refrained from using condoms because of their association with prostitution. In contrast, foreign-born, bordello-based sex workers regarded themselves as "border crossing professionals" who could return home and leave their work in the workplace. As such, they were more likely to use condoms (Kane, 1998).

An additional example of the importance of context and the meaning ascribed to it is provided by findings from interviews conducted with Puerto Rican sex workers in Puerto Rico. The study revealed that, although the women were aware of the possibility of HIV infection due to inconsistent condom use with their primary partners and clients, the threat of HIV was viewed as one of life's many risks that included murder, rape, drug overdose, and assault (Hansen, Lopez-Iftikhar, and Alegría, 2002). Additionally, a number of the women screened their clients to determine which ones did not need to be asked to use a condom; those who were young, clean, attractive, and married were seen as "safe" and "unpolluted." Women who interacted in a more impersonal manner with clients were more likely to refuse to engage in anal or oral sex, while those with more personal, amiable relations with regular clients "extended trust" to clients by forgoing the use of a condom and allowing the clients to pay after, rather than before, sex (Hansen, Lopez-Iftikhar, and Alegría, 2002). Sharing drugs with a client or using drugs in the presence of a client also signaled mutuality and trust, as it left the woman more vulnerable.

Relatively little research has focused on the occurrence of human papillomavirus among sex workers. Those that have have reported the prevalence to be as high as 56% among HIV-positive sex workers in Honduras (Kreiss, Kiviat, Plummer et al., 1992), and as low as 14% among sex workers in Singapore (Ferrera, Belchers, Velema et al., 1997). A study involving 288 commercial sex workers and 266 non-sex worker women attending the same sexual health clinic in Sydney, Australia reported no statistically significant difference in the prevalence of HPV in the two groups of women (Tideman, Thompson, Rose et al., 2003). However, the women employed in sex work had a higher rate of HPV-related cytological abnormalities. HPV infection in both groups was found to be associated with the use of oral contraceptives rather than condoms, an abnormal cervical smear, younger age, and a greater number of non-paying sexual partners (Tideman, Thompson, Rose et al., 2003).

Research indicates that the risk of HIV among male sex workers is significantly associated with sexual orientation. Among male street workers in the U.S., those who self-identify as homosexual are more likely to be HIV-positive than those who are heterosexual or bisexual (Elifson, Boles, and Sweat, 1993; Morse et al., 1991). Male street sex workers who self-identify as gay appear to be more likely to engage in behaviors that carry increased risk, such as serving as the receptive partner during anal sex and engaging in internal water sports, fisting, feces (scat) play, and rimming (Morse et al., 1999). One research group reported that the majority of the sex workers and the majority of the clients did not utilize condoms; the male sex workers reported that police viewed their possession of multiple condoms as evidence that they were engaged in sex work, which would increase the likelihood of their arrest. In addition, it appeared that the majority of heterosexual and homosexual sex workers did not use condoms with their female partners outside of the work environment; many of the partners were sex workers themselves. Consequently, there was an increased risk of HIV transmission outside the work environment as well (Morse et al., 1999).

Although relatively few HIV incidence or prevalence studies have been conducted with male sex workers, the few that exist suggest that HIV prevalence is quite high. In a study of 235 street workers in Atlanta, 29.4% were found to be HIV-positive (Elifson et al., 1993). A study of 211 sex workers in Louisiana reported that 17.5%,or 175 per 1000, were HIV-positive (Morse et al., 1991). These figures indicate a higher prevalence than that found by the Centers for Disease Control among female sex workers, which was 120 per 1000 (Centers for Disease Control, 1987).

Morse and colleagues (1999) reported from their study of 211 male sex workers, that the workers sold more than 164,000 sex acts during a one-year period. Thirty-seven HIV-positive workers reported 30,992 sexual contacts in a year, or 2.3 encounters per day per person. The vast majority of the 211 workers perceived HIV/AIDS as very serious and believed that they had more than a 50% chance of contracting it.

Davies and Feldman (1999) found that male sex workers may engage in a wide range of behaviors that includes masturbation, oral sex, S&M activity such as spanking, and anal sex. Frequently, those who did not use a condom did so because they were threatened with violence. Condom use was found to be more common with casual, as compared with regular, partners.

As with female sex workers, the context in which the sex work occurs may be critical to understanding the level of risk and the (un)willingness of the sex worker to accept a certain level of risk. For instance, the work environment of male sex workers who utilize the internet differs in significant ways from that of the street-based male sex worker. Internet workers can work from their own homes, can screen their prospective clients prior to meeting them, can set their own fees and negotiate their own terms, and can retain their earnings (Gaffney, 2003, cited in Parsons, Koken, and Bimbi, 2004). One study with 46 internet-based gay and bisexual male sex workers found that less than half reported unprotected anal sex with clients, while the majority refused to engage in any unsafe sexual practices. In addition, many used their encounters with their clients as an opportunity to explain the risks associated with unprotected sex (Parsons, Koken, and Bimbi, 2004). Those who refused requests for unprotected sex often lost the prospective client, but indicated that the immediate financial reward was not worth the potential long-term cost. The majority of these men were white, gay men who had a college degree; 20% had completed some graduate-level coursework. These characteristics may distinguish them in critical ways from the majority of male street-based sex workers who lack their level of education and may, as a result, possess fewer available internal and external resources that support them in their efforts to reduce risk (Morse, Simon, Osofsky, Balson, and Gaumer, 1991; Weber, Craib, Chan et al., 2001).

Individuals who are forced through trafficking to engage in sex work may face heightened risk. In interviews with women who had been trafficked and forced to work as sex workers in Europe, many of the women reported having 10 to 25 clients per night, while some women were forced to service as many as 50 per night (Zimmerman, Yun, Schvab et al., 2003). Almost one-quarter of the women interviewed indicated that condoms were not used regularly for vaginal sex and more than half of the women did not use condoms when they had sexual relations with their pimp or intimate partners. All of the women reported that they had been sexually abused, forced to commit sexual acts involuntarily, including unprotected oral and anal sex, and had been gang raped (Zimmerman, Yun, Schvab et al., 2003).

Similar circumstances were found in interviews with brothel-based sex workers from eastern Europe, most of whom had been voluntarily trafficked from their countries of origin to Israel. Although all of the women reported using condoms for vaginal sex, none had used condoms for oral sex (Chudakov, Ilan, Belmaker, and Cwikel, 2002). The women provide services to an average of 12 clients per day, although some had as many as 25 per day. Almost half reported that they worked throughout the month, including during menstruation. Limited data from this same study suggest that there may be significant differences between trafficked women who obtain legal residence in the destination country and those who do not. Those with legal resident status tended to be older, to have started sex work at a later age, to work fewer hours per day and fewer days per week, and did not work while menstruating (Cwikel, Ilan, and Chudakov, 2003). Although it was unclear whether these same conditions prevailed when the women first began sex work, their reduced work hours and concomitant reduction in the number of clients may have helped to reduce their risk of exposure to sexually transmitted disease.

Although the incidence and prevalence of sexually transmitted infections among those who work in the pornography industry are not known, it appears that the risks are quite high. As previously indicated, an actor/model may have between 24 and 32 different sexual partners each month in the course of work alone and may have multiple encounters with each; each of these individuals have had, in turn, encounters with as many as 23 to 31 other partners. The majority of these work-related sexual encounters are without the benefit of condoms or other safer sex strategies. Even in 1986, five years into the HIV/AIDS epidemic, HIV/AIDS had done little to change the practices within the industry, as evidenced by an interview of Amber Lynn, a leading porn star, by *Hustler*:

Hustler: You're f...ing so many men these days, aren't you afraid of AIDS? Many actors in the business are bisexual.
Amber: There's an incredible fear of AIDS sweeping through the X-rated-film business right now. All of my girlfriends are talking about it. We're scared to death that we'll find out in three years we've only got a few months left.
Hustler: Why do you continue your promiscuous career then?
Amber: I get a blood test regularly and am very careful about the people I work with. Hey, life's a f...ing gamble anyway, and there is where I want to be. I can't think of doing anything else. That's not to say I'm reckless. For instance, I won't f... some guy I know has been f...ing a bunch of other guys not for a lousy thousand dollars. It's not worth it to me, because if I get AIDS, then everyone I come in contact with [will] get it and not just the people I work with, but the people I love and care about too (Amber Lynn, 1986: 24, 30).

Mental Health

Relatively little empirical research has been conducted to examine the mental health effects of voluntary commercial partnering. It has been asserted that prostitution itself serves to objectify women: "A person is sexually objectified when her sexual parts or sexual functions are separated out from the rest of her personality and reduced to the status of mere instruments or else regarded as if they were capable of representing her . . . . (Bartky, 1990: 26). This theoretical assertion has not, however, been subjected to vigorous testing. In addition, this writer was unable to locate any studies relating to the mental health effects of participating as the paying partner in voluntary commercial partnering.

Interviews with 47 female sex workers in Canada found that many engaged in cutting behavior in order to reduce or eliminate the pain associated with the violence that others inflicted on them (Nixon, Tutty, Downe, Gorkoff, and Ursel, 2003). Almost one-fifth of the women had attempted suicide.

In contrast, Zuilhof (1999) found in his research with male sex workers in the Netherlands that many used their work as an opportunity to experiment with their own sexuality and sexual identity. Many times, they derived a sense of belonging when they shared their accommodations with other males engaged in the same work. Clients, or sugar daddies, often assumed the role of informal social workers and attempted to assist the young workers.

The mental health consequences of being trafficked have not been systematically assessed (Gazi et al., 2001; International Organization for Migration, 1996). Interviews with a small number of primarily involuntarily trafficked women indicate that the travel and transit stage of trafficking may provoke acute anxiety, resulting in difficulties with memory at a later time and consequent difficulties recounting the details of their circumstances to authorities (Zimmerman, Yun, Schvab et al., 2003). Women who are trafficked may often blame themselves for their circumstances, feeling that they should have recognized the deceptive tactics that were used or made successful efforts to escape. These feelings of guilt may result in lowered self-esteem and feelings of distrust.

While under the control of their traffickers at the destination stage, women were often subjected to psychological tactics that were designed to manipulate them, including intimidation, threats, lies, and the imposition of unsafe and unpredictable events. As a result, many of the women reported fatigue, frequent headaches, frequent sadness, and feelings of worthlessness. A number of individuals also reported thoughts about suicide (Zimmerman, Yun, Schvab et al., 2003). Interviews with previously trafficked women indicate that, due to the stigma associated with commercial sex work, some women who have been trafficked may have to turn to prostitution to support themselves upon their return to their home countries (Foundation of Women's Forum, 1998).

An interview-based study with 55 trafficked women in Israel, most of whom had been voluntarily trafficked with knowledge that they would be engaging in sex work, similarly reported a high prevalence of mental health concerns (Chudakov, Ilan, Belmaker, and Cwikel, 2002). Almost one-fifth of the women evidenced symptoms of posttraumatic stress disorder (PTSD), one-third had depressive symptoms, and almost one-fifth were clinically depressed. Twenty-three of the 55 women had experienced abuse as children and had suffered physical violence and rape during sex work. A history of past trauma was found to be associated with the initiation of sex work at a younger age and symptoms of PTSD (Chudakov, Ilan, Belmaker, and Cwikel, 2002).

It has been asserted that pornography directly harms women who work in the pornography industry through violence, degradation, and sexual abuse (cf. Cole, 1989) and causes harm to women through its promulgation of negative attitudes towards and beliefs about women (Lacombe, 1994). These assertions were echoed by William Margold, described by the Attorney General's Commission on Pornography (1986) as a "leading figure" in the adult film industry, who advised the Commission:

And I'd like to point out that for a woman, there's even more of a stigma than for a man. She'll be called a prostitute and a whore and thought of as sleazy, cheap and slutty. And she has to understand that what she does now will haunt her the rest of her life.

The mental health consequences of participating in the production of pornographic videos and films have not been systematically investigated. Research has suggested that exposure to pornography activates sexually callous perceptions of women and promotes sexually aggressive behavior by men (Weaver, 1992). A meta-analysis of experimental studies found that even material that depicts nonviolent sexual activity increases aggressive behavior and depictions of violent sexual activity produce even greater aggression (Allen, D'Alessio, and Brezgel, 1995). It is not known whether these same findings would hold true for those who have participated in the production of the pornography, as distinct from the viewing, or whether the effects might be even more extreme.

Substance Use

Substance use, violence, sex work, and HIV risk often go hand in hand. In-depth interviews with 35 women participating in a study of HIV risk among out-of-treatment drug users in Hartford, Connecticut revealed that the women had few economic opportunities not only because of their substance use, but also because of their low levels of education and, in some cases, limited English proficiency (Romero-Daza, Weeks, and Singer, 2003). Most had begun using drugs in their teens in an effort to fit in with their peers and/or as a means of dealing with the physical and verbal abuse that they suffered in their homes. Those who began drug use as adults did so in an attempt to alleviate the stress caused by partner violence. Many of the women witnessed extreme violence on the streets, leading to intensified drug use in an effort to drown out their emotional pain (Romero-Daza, Weeks, and Singer, 2003).

Research with male street sex workers suggests that polysubstance use is normative (Morse et al., 1999). Liguori and Aggleton (1999) have found that male sex workers may also use drugs to reduce the fear that they feel on the street, while others may utilize substances while they are engaged in sex work. Consequently, impaired decisionmaking may contribute to the absence of safer sex precautions. Those who inject drugs are at additional risk of HIV transmission as a result of their sharing of injection equipment with their clients, other sex workers, and non-work partners (Morse et al., 1999). Somewhat counterintuitively, it has also been found that the frequent use of substances in conjunction with male sex work may decrease the incidence of high risk behavior by causing a disinterest in sexual activity and sex work (Morse et al., 1999). This suggests that those who engage in the highest levels of risk are the least likely to engage in polysubstance use.

Women who have been the victims of trafficking have reported being forced to use drugs or alcohol in order to be able to take on more clients, work longer hours, or perform objectionable acts (Zimmerman, Yun, Schvab et al., 2003). While the prevalence of substance use within the pornography industry is unknown, at least some of the actors/models use substances in order to do their work. One woman testified to the Attorney General's Commission on Pornography that she used drugs because "you have to hide, you have to keep your feelings and emotions from being completely destroyed. Each day [in the industry] erodes them away"(Attorney General's Commission on Pornography, 1986).

Violent and Nonviolent Injury

Rosen (1982) found from her study of U.S. sex workers and their environment during the early twentieth century that the levels of violence against commercial sex workers increased following the disappearance of red light districts. Violence from clients and pimps is not unusual (Edward, 1993; Hoigard and Finstad, 1991; McKegany and Bernard, 1996; McLeod, 1982; Romero-Daza, Weeks, and Singer, 2003). Women who work on the streets may also suffer violence at the hands of drug users, who need money or drugs (Romero-Daza, Weeks, and Singer, 2003). A study of adolescent and child prostitution in Los Angeles identified violence as a common theme among the sex workers; the violence often took the form of rape, torture, slavery, and murder (Nicholsen, 1981).

For many women engaged in sex work, violence is a normative experience, beginning with childhood physical and sexual abuse and extending into adulthood. A focus group-base study conducted with 325 crack- and heroin-using sex workers in Miami found that almost one-half had experienced physical abuse during childhood and one-half had suffered childhood sexual abuse. During the previous year, one-quarter had been beaten and almost one-half had encountered a violent client (Surratt, Inciardi, Kurts, and Kiley, 2004). Fully one-quarter of 35 female sex workers participating in a focus group-based study in Hartford, Connecticut reported having had friends who were murdered while selling sex (Romero-Daza, Weeks, and Singer, 2003). Such murders of female sex workers are most frequently caused by one male (Liguori and Aggleton, 1999), in contrast to the injury or murder of male sex workers, who are more likely to be attacked by a group of men intent on maximizing the brutality of their attack (Liguori and Aggleton, 1999).

Violence has been found to be a common risk associated with commercial sex work in countries outside of the U.S. as well (Foundation of Women's Forum, 1998). An interview study with 47 women engaged in legal sex work in three western Canadian provinces found that one-half had been threatened with or had suffered violence from pimps while engaged in sex work and more than one-half had experienced violence from their clients (Nixon, Tutty, Downe, Gorkoff, and Ursel, 2002). Assaults included stabbings, rape, gang rape, beating, choking, torture, and being run over; injuries often resulted in hospitalization. Almost one-fourth had been coerced into prostitution by their boyfriends. More than three-quarters of the women had suffered sexual abuse as a child; violence experienced in the context of sex work was normative and the women had become desensitized to it. Many feared violence at the hands of the police and the general public (Nixon, Tutty, Downe, Gorkoff, and Ursel, 2002).

In yet another study, also conducted in Canada, a review of medical records of an emergency department assault service found that most of the 96 female sex workers who had been sexually assaulted suffered injuries as a result of the assault (DuMont and McGregor, 2004). Compared to the 366 other women whose medical records were also examined, the sex workers were more likely to be younger and to be users of heroin and/or cocaine.

Individuals who are trafficked for the purpose of voluntary sex work or involuntary sexual exploitation may be subject to violence as a means of establishing control over them. Individuals who have been trafficked have reported suffering broken bones, contusions, pain, loss of consciousness, and headaches due to the intentional infliction of injury on them by their captors (Zimmerman, Yun, Schvab et al., 2003). Of 55 women, most of whom were voluntarily trafficked to Israel for brothel-based sex work, 31% were threatened, 15% were threatened with a gun, 30% were physically assaulted at work, and 30% were sexually assaulted at work (Cwikel, Ilan, and Chudakov, 2003). Vulnerability is likely heightened due to individuals' social and legal isolation and their lack of access to supportive resources (Anon., 1999; Gushulak & MacPherson, 2000).

A study of women trafficked in Europe yielded similar findings. The 28 women interviewed in the study originated from seven different countries and were trafficked to 11 different destination countries (Zimmerman et al., 2003). Twenty-five of the 28 were forced into sex work. Thirty-five percent suffered physical violence prior to their departure from their home countries, almost 90% experienced physical violence during the trafficking, and all of the women were subjected to sexual abuse and coercion during the trafficking experience (Zimmerman et al., 2003). One woman recounted how she had been trafficked and then through deception and violence forced to participate in sex work:

A friend offered to help me leave [the Ukraine] for a nanny job in the UK. I accepted. Damek arranged my documents and travel to the UK. When we arrived at the border, I changed my mind about going. Damek slapped me and made me continue on; he said that he could kill me. In London, Damek told me that I would be working as a prostitute and he raped me to show me that I would have no choice . . . . (Zimmerman, 2004: 565).

The frequency and severity of nonviolent injury in the context of trafficking is likely related to the mode of transportation that is used during the travel and transit stage (Zimmerman, Yun, Schvab et al., 2003). Trafficked persons are often concealed in goods or cargo; falls from the conveyance or exposure to the cargo can result in serious injury or death (BBC World Service, 1999). Persons who are trafficked in containers or trunks may be deprived of adequate air, water, and/or nutrition, leading to injury or death (Veronneau, Mohler, Pennybaker et al., 1996). Those trafficked by ship face the possibility of infectious disease transmission due to unsanitary conditions (Solitar, Lozada, Tseng et al., 1998) or suffocation (Ha, 1999). Illegal desert crossings, such as those between Mexico and the southern border of the U.S., can result in dehydration, high-elevation cold, and/or death (Gross, 1999a, 1999b). Attempts to evade legal authorities during trafficking often involve dangerous activities, such as high speed car chases, that can lead to serious injury and death (Walker, 1999).

Child Development

Almost no literature exists that examines the impact of a parent's sex work on child development or the mental health of children. This may be due, in large part, to the removal of many children by child protective services from homes in which one or both of the parents engage in sex work. Women often recognize that their commercial sex work may be detrimental to their child (Nixon, Tutty, Downe, Gorkoff, and Ursel, 2003), but may see few available alternative means to support their children (Hansen, Lopez-Ifitkhar, and Alegría, 2002).

Implications for Research and Practice

Relatively little research has focused on the health implications of commercial partnering in any form, aside from investigations related to sexually transmitted infections including, in particular, HIV/AIDS. Even these studies have focused, for the most part, on disease transmission within the context of seemingly voluntary commercial sex work, to the exclusion of additional dimensions, such as sex work resulting from forced trafficking, forced work conditions following voluntary trafficking, or participation in adult pornography.

Ultimately, this lack of knowledge impedes our ability to develop effective interventions, that may or may not be directly health-related, that positively impact health. For instance, economic interventions could presumably disrupt the existing economic equilibrium in a particular locality. Without an adequate understanding of the economic factors that have contributed to the decisionmaking and actions of the traffickers, those who have been trafficked, those who utilize the services of the trafficked individuals, and those who may benefit more indirectly from the trafficking, it would be difficult, if not impossible, to formulate an effective economic intervention to reduce or eliminate trafficking and, indirectly, the adverse health effects of trafficking.

Because researchers often use the same words to mean different things and fail to define specifically the concept to which their words refer, it is often difficult to compare research findings and, ultimately to draw conclusions from the research that is done. This confusion has serious implications for the formulation of policy that is founded on published research; those responsible for the formulation of legislation and regulations may or may not have insight into the underlying confusion, depending upon their level of familiarity with the research.

The assumptions that underlie many of our policies related to commercial partnering may inadvertently erect barriers to the search for and provision of health-related services. Individuals who have been or perceive that they have been stigmatized because of their activities, whether engaged in on a voluntary or involuntary basis, may be less willing to seek needed services when they are able to do so as a result of shame, embarrassment, and fear. Providers who have failed to examine and address their own assumptions and values as they relate to commercial partnering may unknowingly hamper communication by their client or patient. For instance, providers who mistakenly believe that all trafficked persons are transported against their will may inadvertently foreclose the possibility of exploring with their patient-client emotional trauma that was associated with a decision to seek the assistance of a known trafficker.

References

Aggleton, P. (Ed.). (1999). *Men Who Sell Sex*. Philadelphia: Temple University Press.

Agocs, M.M., Trent, R.B., Russell, D.M. (1994). Activities associated with drownings in Imperial County, CA, 1980-90: Implications for prevention. *Public Health Reports* 109: 290-295.

Albert, A. (2001). *Brothel: Mustang Ranch and Its Women*. New York: Random House.

Ali, S. (1998). *Trafficking in Children and Their Commercial Sexual Exploitation in Prostitution and Other Intolerable Forms of Child Labour in Bangladesh: Country Report.* Dhaka: Bangladesh National Women Lawyers' Association.

Allen, M., D'Alessio, D., Brezgel, K. (1995). A meta-analysis summarizing the effects of pornography. II. Aggression after exposure. *Human Communication Research* 22: 258-283.

Allen, M., Emmers, T.M., Gebhardt, L., Giery, M.A. (1995). Exposure to pornography and acceptance of rape myths. Journal of Communication 45: 5-26.

Allen, R.E. (Ed.). (1990). *Concise Oxford Dictionary of Current English,* 8th ed. Oxford: Clarendon Press.

Altink, S. (1995). *Stolen Lives: Trading Women into Sex and Slavery.* New York: Harrington Park Press.

Amber Lynn: Porn's busiest beaver.(1986). *Hustler,* April: 24, 30.

Anon. (1998). Europe, Italy, Spain: Illegal immigrants, Spain. *Migration News* 5(10). Available at http://migration.ucdavis.edu.

Anon. (1999). Five arrested in teens' deaths. Police say two Canadians killed by their U.S. escort agency bodyguards. *Hamilton Spectator* August 7: D12.

Archivantikul, K. (1998). Trafficking in Children for Labour Exploitation including Child Prostitution in the Mekong Sub-Region (dissertation). Bangkok, Thailand: Institute for Population and Social Research, Mahidol University.

Associated Press. (1999). 40 Haitians presumed dead in Florida boat sinkings. March.

Attorney General's Commission on Pornography. (1986). *Final Report.* July. Washington, D.C.: United States Department of Justice. Available at http://www.porn-report.com. Last accessed March 24, 2005.

Bartky, S. (1990). *Femininity and Domination: Studies in the Phenomenology of Oppression.* New York: Routledge.

BBC World Service. (1999). Six die in Spanish ships hold, October 2. Available at http://news2bbc.co.uk/hi/english/world/europenewsid%5F463000/463720.stm.

Boseman, J., Ross, M., Williams, M. (1999). Sale of sex for drugs and drugs for sex: An economic context of sexual risk behaviors for STDs. *Sexually Transmitted Diseases* 26(8): 444-449.

Bruch, E.M. (2004). Models wanted: The search for an effective response to human trafficking. *Stanford Journal of International Law* 40: 1-45.

Bullough, V.L., Bullough, B.L. (1964). *The History of Prostitution.* New Hyde Park, New York: University Press.

Caulkins, S.E., Coombs, N.R. (1976). The psychodynamics of male prostitution. *American Journal of Psychotherapy* 30: 441-451.

Centers for Disease Control and Prevention. (1987). Antibody to human immunodeficiency virus in female prostitutes. *Morbidity & Mortality Weekly Report* 36: 157-161.

Chudakov, B., Ilan, K., Belmaker, R.H., Cwikel, J. (2002). The motivation and mental health of sex workers. *Journal of Sex & Marital Therapy* 28: 305-315.

Cole, S.G. (1989). *Pornography and the Sex Crises.* Toronto: Amanita Enterprises.

Cwikel, J., Chudakov, B., Paikin, M., Agmon, K., Belmaker, R.H. (2004). Trafficked female sex workers awaiting deportation: Comparison with brothel workers. *Archives of Women's Mental Health* 7: 243-249.

Cwikel, J., Ilan, K., Chudakov, B. (2003). Women brothel workers and occupational health risks. *Journal of Epidemiology and Community Health* 57(10): 809-815.

Davies, P.M., Feldman, R. (1991). Selling sex in Cardiff and London. In P. Aggleton, P.M. Davies, G. Hart (Eds.), *AIDS: Individual, Cultural and Policy Dimensions* (pp. 1-22). London: Falmer Press.

Davies, P.M., Simpson, P. (1990). On male homosexual prostitution and HIV. In P. Aggleton, P.M. Davies, G. Hart (Eds.), *AIDS: Individual, Cultural and Policy Dimensions.* London: Falmer Press.

Davis, N.J. (2000). From victims to survivors: Working with recovering street prostitutes. In R. Weitzer (Ed.), *Sex for Sale: Prostitution, Pornography, and the Sex Industry* (pp. 139-158). New York: Routledge.

Dietz, P.E., Evans, B. (1982). Pornographic imagery and prevalence of paraphilia. *American Journal of Psychiatry* 139: 1493-1495.

Donnerstein, E., Berkowitz, L. (1981). Victim reactions in aggressive erotic films as a factor in violence against women. *Journal of Personalities and Social Psychology* 41: 710-724.

Donnerstein, E., Berkowitz, L. (1986). Mass media sexual violence and male viewers: Current theory and research. *American Behavioral Scientists* 29: 601-618.

DuMont, J., McGregor, M.J. (2004). Sexual assault in the lives of urban sex workers: A descriptive and comparative analysis. *Women & Health* 39(3): 79-96.

Elifson, K.W., Boles, J., Sweat, M. (1993). Risk factors associated with HIV infection among male prostitutes. *American Journal of Public Health* 83: 79-83.

Falck, R.S., Wang, J., Carlson, R.G., Siegel, H.A. (2001). The epidemiology of physical attack and rape among crack-using women. Violence and Victims 16(1): 79-89.

Ferrera, A., Belchers, W.J.G., Velema, J.P., Figueroa, M. (1997). Association of infections with human immunodeficiency virus and human papillomavirus in Honduras. *American Journal of Tropical Medicine & Hygiene* 57(2): 138-141.

Fisher, W.A., Barak, A. (1991). Pornography, erotica, and behavior: More questions than answers. *International Journal of Law & Psychiatry* 14: 65-83.

Foundation of Women's Forum/Stiftelsen Kvinnoforum. (1998). Trafficking in Women for the Purpose of Sexual Exploitation: Mapping the Situation and Existing Organisations in Baelarus, Russia, the Baltic and Nordic States. Stockholm, Sweden: Foundation of Women's Forum/Stiftelsen Kvinnoforum. Available at http://www.qweb.kvinnoforum.se/papers/traffickingreport.html. Last accessed March 12, 2005.

Gaffney, J. (2003). Working together with male sex workers (MSW) in London. Paper presented at the European Network of Male Prostitution, Hamburg, German.

Gazi, R., Chowdhury, Z.H., Alam, S.M.N., Chowdhury, E., Ahmed, F., Begum, S. (2001). *Trafficking of Women and Children in Bangladesh:*

An Overview. Dhaka, Bangladesh: ICDDR,B: Centre for Health and Population Research.

Gilbert, L., El-Bassel, N., Rajah, V., Foleno, A., Frye, V. (2001). Linking drug-related activities with experiences of partner violence: A focus group study of women in methadone treatment. *Violence and Victims* 16(5): 517-536.

Gross, G.A. (1999a). Bodies of two men found in Imperial Valley desert. *San Diego Union Tribune* Sept. 8: B-3.

Gross, G.A. (1999b). Five-year old Gatekeeper is praised, denounced. Critics say it makes border more dangerous. *San Diego Union Tribune* Oct. 31: B-1.

Gushulak, B., MacPherson, D.W. (2000). Health issues associated with the smuggling and trafficking of migrants. *Journal of Immigrant Health* 2(2): 67-78.

Ha, T.T. (1999). Three stowaways suffocated, autopsies find. The Globe and Mail, April 21. Available at http://www.theglobeandmail.com/gam/National/19990421/UREWFUM.html.

Hansen, H., Lopez-Iftikhar, M.M., Alegría, M. (2002). Economy of risk and respect: Accounts by Puerto Rican sex workers of HIV risk taking. *The Journal of Sex Research* 39(4): 292-301.

Harsanyi, D.P. (1993). Women in Romania. In N. Funk, M. Mueller (Eds.). *Gender, Politics, and Post-Communism* (pp. 39-52). New York: Routledge.

Hoigard, C., Finstad, L. (1992). *Backstreets: Money, Prostitution and Love.* Cambridge,U.K.: Polity Press.

International Organization for Migration. (2003). *Irregular Migration and Trafficking in Women: The Case of Turkey.* Brussels: Author. Available at http://www.ion.int/iomwebsite/Publication/ServletSearchPublication?event=detail&id=2871. Last accessed March 12, 2005.

International Organisation for Migration. (2001). New global figures on the global scale of trafficking. *Trafficking in Migrants Bulletin,* 23. Available at http://www.iom.int//documents/publications/en/tm_23.pdf. Last accessed February 2002.

International Organisation for Migration. (1999). *Trafficking in Migrants. IOM Policy and Responses.* Brussels: Author.

International Organization for Migration. (1996). *Trafficking in Women to Austria for Sexual Exploitation.* Brussels: Author.

Kane, S. (1998). *AIDS Alibis: Sex, Drugs, and Crime in the Americas.* Philadelphia: Temple University Press.

Khan, Z.R., Arefeen, H.K. (1988). *Polita nari—A Study of Prostitution in Bangladesh.* Dhaka, Bangladesh: Centre for Social Studies, Dhaka University.

Kreiss, J., Kiviat, N., Plummer, F.A., Roberts, P.L., Waiyaki, P., Ngugi, E., Holmes, K.K. (1992). Human immunodeficiency virus, human papillomavirus and cervical intraepithelial neoplasia in Nairobi prostitutes. *Sexually Transmitted Disease* 19(1): 54-58.

Lacombe, D. (1994). *Blue Politics: Pornography and Law in the Age of Feminism.* Toronto, Canada: University of Toronto Press.

Laws, D.R., Marshall, W.L. (1990). A conditioning theory of the etiology and maintenance of deviant sexual preference and behavior. In W.L. Marshall, D.R. Laws, H.E. Barbaree (Eds.), *Handbook of Sexual Assault: Issues, Theories, and Treatment of the Offender* (pp. 209-229). New York: Plenum Press.

Liguori, A.L., Aggleton, P. (1999). Aspects of male sex work in Mexico City. In P. Aggleton, P.M. Davies, G. Hart (Eds.), *AIDS: Individual, Cultural and Policy Dimensions* (pp. 103-125). London: Falmer Press.

Linz, D., Donnerstein, E., Penrod, S. (1984). The effects of multiple exposures to films violence against women. *Journal of Communication* 34: 130-147.

Linz, D., Donnerstein, E., Penrod, S. (1987). Sexual violence in the mass media: Social psychological implications. In P. Shaver, C. Hendrick (Eds.), *Review of Personality and Social Psychology: Vol. 7: Sex and Gender* (pp. 95-123). Newbury Park, California: Sage.

MacKinnon, C.A. (1987). *Feminism Unmodified: Discourses on Life and Law.* Cambridge: Harvard University Press.

Marshall, W.L., Barrett, S. (1990). *Criminal Neglect: Why Sex Offenders Go Free.* Toronto: Doubleday.

McDonald, L., Moore, B., Timoshkina, N. (2000). *Migrant Sex Workers from Eastern Europe and the Former Soviet Union: The Canadian Case.* Toronto, Canada: Centre for Applied Social Research, University of Toronto.

McKegany, N., Bernard, M. (1996). *Sex Work on the Streets*. Buckingham: Open University Press.

McLeod, E. (1982). *Women Working: Prostitution Now*. London: Croom Helm.

Miller v. California. (1972). 413 U.S. 15.

Morse, E.V., Simon, P.M., Burchfiel, K.E. (1999). Social environment and male sex work in the United States. In P. Aggleton (Ed.)., *Men Who Sell Sex* (pp. 83-101). Philadelphia: Temple University Press

Morse, E.V., Simon, P.M., Osofsky, H.J., Balson, P.M., Gaumer, H.R. (1991). The male street prostitute: A vector for transmission of HIV infection into the heterosexual world. *Social Science & Medicine* 32: 535-539.

Nagi, B.S. (1993). *Child Marriage in India*. New Delhi, India: Mittal Publications.

Nicholsen, A.H. (1981). *Youth in Crisis: A Study of Adolescent and Child Prostitution*. Los Angeles, California: Gay and Lesbian Community Services Center.

Nixon, K., Tutty, L., Downe, P., Gorkoff, K., Ursel, J. (2003). The everyday occurrence: Violence in the lives of girls exploited through prostitution. *Violence Against Women* 8(9): 1016-1043.

O'Neill, M. (2001). *Prostitution & Feminism: Towards a Politics of Feeling*. Oxford, U.K.: Blackwell Publishers Limited.

O'Neill, R.A. (1999). *International Trafficking in Women to the United States: A Contemporary Manifestation of Slavery and Organized Crime*. Washington, D.C.: Center for the Study of Intelligence. Available at http://www.cia.gov/csi/monograph/women/trafficking.pdf. Last accessed May 5, 2000).

Parsons, J.T., Koken, J.A., Bimbi, D.S. (2004). The use of the internet by gay and bisexual male escorts: Sex workers as sex educators. *AIDS Care* 16(8): 1021-1035.

Peterson, J.R. (1995). In the rules of the game. *Playboy*, October.

Rabjhandari, R., Rabjhandari, J. (1997). *Girl Trafficking: The Hidden Grief in the Himalayas*. Nepal: WOREC.

Romero-Daza, N., Weeks, M., Singer, M. (2003). "Nobody gives a damn if I live or die": Violence, drugs, and street-level prostitution in inner-city Hartford, Connecticut. *Medical Anthropology* 22: 233-259.

Rosen, R. (1982). *The Lost Sisterhood: Prostitution in America, 1900-1918*. Baltimore: Johns Hopkins University Press.

Seto, M.C., Maric, A., Barbaree, H.E. (2001). The role of pornography in the etiology of sexual aggression. *Aggression and Violent Behavior* 6: 35-53.

Solitar, B.M., Lozada, C.J., Tseng, C.E., Lowe, A.M., Krajewski, W.M., Blanchard, K., Pillinger, M., Weissman, G., Weismann, G. (1998). Reiter's syndrome: Asian ship-board immigrants: The case of the Golden Venture. *Seminars in Arthritis and Rheumatology* 27: 293-300.

Steinfatt, T.M. (2000). *Working at the Bar*. Westport, Connecticut: Ablex Publishing.

Stetson, D.B. (2004). The invisible issue: Prostitution and trafficking of women and girls in the United States. In J. Outshoorn, (Ed.), *The Politics of Prostitution: Women's Movements, Democratic States and the Globalisation of Sex Commerce* (pp. 245-264). Cambridge, U.K.: Cambridge University Press.

Surratt, H.L., Inciardi, J.A., Kurtz, S.P., Kiley, M.C. (2004). Sex work and drug use in a subculture of violence. *Crime & Delinquency* 50(1): 43-59.

Tideman, R.L., Thompson, C., Rose, B., Gilmour, S., Marks, C., van Beek, I., Berry, G., O'Connor, C., Mindel, A. (2003). Cervical human papillomavirus infections in commercial sex workers—risk factors and behaviours. *International Journal of STD & AIDS* 14: 840-847.

United Nations Office for Drug Control and Crime Prevention. (2000). The Protocol to Prevent, Suppress, and Punish Trafficking in Persons, Especially Women and Children. Available at http://odccp.org//trafficking_protocol.html. Last accessed February, 2002.

Veronneau, S.J., Mohler, S.R., Pennybaker, A.L., Wilcox, B.C., Sahiar, F. (1996). Survival at high altitudes: Wheel-well passengers. *Aviation, Space, Environmental Medicine* 67(8): 784-786.

Victims of Trafficking and Violence Protection Act. (2000). Pub. L. No. 106-386, Div. A; 114 Stat. 1464, Oct. 28.

Walker, S.L. (1999). Deadly crossing: The crash that killed Border Patrol agent Stephen Sullivan and three migrants provokes troubling questions on both sides of the border. *San Diego Union Tribune* August 1: A-1.

Weaver, J. (1992). The Social science and psychological research evidence: Perceptual and behavioral consequences of exposure to pornography. In C. Itzen (Ed.), *Pornography: Women, Violence, and Civil Liberties* (pp. 236-247). Oxford: Oxford University Press.

Weber, A.E., Craib, K.J., Chan, K., Martindale, S., Miller, M.L., Schechter, M.T., Hogg, R.S. (2001). Sex trade involvement and rates of human immunodeficiency virus positivity among young gay and bisexual men. *International Journal of Epidemiology* 30(6): 1449-1454.

Wennerholm, C.J. (2002). Crossing borders and building bridges: The Baltic Region Networking Project. In R. Masika (Ed.), *Gender, Trafficking, and Slavery*. Oxford, England: Oxfam.

Wenzel, S.L., Leake, BD., Gelberg, L. (2001). Risk factors for major violence among homeless women. *Journal of Interpersonal Violence* 16(8): 739-752.

Women's Publishing House and Media Resource Organization. (1998). *Efforts to Prevent Trafficking in Women and Girls: A Pre-Study for Media Activism.* Kathmandu: ASMITA.

Zillmann, D., Bryant, J. (1982). Pornography, sexual callousness, and the trivialization of rape. *Journal of Communication* 32: 10-21.

Zillmann, D., Bryant, J. (1984). Effects of massive exposure to pornography. In N. Malamuth, E. Donerstein (Eds.), *Pronography and Sexual Aggression* (pp. 115-138). Orlando, Florida: Academic Press.

Zimmerman, C. (2004). Risks and responsibilities: Guidelines for interviewing trafficked women. *Lancet* 363: 565.

Zimmerman, C., Yun, K., Schvab, I., Watts, C., Trappolin, L., Treppete, M. et al. (2003). The Health Risks and Consequences of Trafficking in Women and Adolescents. Findings from a European Study. London: London School of Hygiene & Tropical Medicine (LSHTM). Available at http://www.lshtm.ac.uk/hpu/docs/traffickingfinal.pdf. Last accessed March 12, 2005.

Zuilhof, W. (1999). Sex for money between men and boys in the Netherlands: Implications for HIV prevention. In P. Aggleton, P.M. Davies, G. Hart (Eds.), *AIDS: Individual, Cultural and Policy Dimensions* (pp. 23-29). London: Falmer Press.

CHAPTER 5

Object Relations: Fetish And Related Behaviors

Defining Fetish

Unlike other chapters of this book that focus on partnering between two or more people and the health effects of such partnerings, this chapter focuses on attraction to objects and/or anatomical portions of people and related health effects. In effect, at the extreme, the attraction to the object becomes the relationship with the object. This may occur regardless of the sex or sexual orientation of the individuals involved.

The nature and cause of fetish sexual practice has been the subject of vociferous debate. *Webster's Third New International Dictionary Unabridged* (1986) defines a fetish as a

natural or artificial object (as an animal tooth or a wood carving) believed among a primitive people to have a preternatural power to protect or aid its owner often because of ritual consecration or animation by a spirit; broadly: any material object regarded with superstitious or extravagant trust or reverence.

Fire, for instance, can be the object of such a fetish (Balachandra, 2002).

The nineteenth-century sexologist Krafft-Ebing (1886: 218) used the term fetishism to refer to "The Association of Lust with the Idea of Certain Portions of the Female Person, or with Certain Articles of Female Attire." Krafft-Ebing postulated that pathological erotic

153

fetishism occurred when "the fetich itself (rather than the person associated with it) becomes the exclusive object of sexual desire" so that, rather than sexual intercourse, "strange manipulations of the fetich" became the sexual aim (Krafft-Ebing, 1886; spelling as in original text). Empirical research, however, suggests that intimacy and fetishism are able to coexist, either within a specific relationship, or through the maintenance of a primary relationship while engaging in fetish behavior with outside partners (Weinberg, Williams, and Calhan, 1994).

The intensity of fetishism has been conceived of as existing on a spectrum, as follows (Gamman and Makinen, 1994: 38).

Level 1: Individuals experience a slight preference for certain kinds of sex partners, sexual stimuli or sexual activity. The term "fetish" should not be applied at this level.

Level 2: This represents the lowest level of fetishism, where a strong preference exists for certain kinds of sex partners, sexual stimuli or sexual activity.

Level 3: At this level, fetishism is moderately intense and individuals require specific stimuli in order to experience sexual arousal and perform sexually.

Level 4: This level represents the highest level of fetishism, where specific stimuli take the place of a sex partner.

Fetishism is also conceived of as a mental disorder. The current reference work for the diagnosis of mental disorders, the *Diagnostic and Statistical Manual, Fourth Edition, Text Revision* (DSM-IV-TR, 2000) classifies *fetishism* as a paraphilia and sets forth diagnostic criteria for what is considered to be a disorder: recurrent, intense sexually arousing sexual fantasies, sexual urges, or behaviors involving the use of nonliving objects for a period of at least six months; clinically significant distress or impairment in social, occupational, or other important areas of functioning as a result of these fantasies, urges, or behaviors; and the nonliving objects consist of articles beyond the use of female clothing used in cross-dressing or devices designed for the purpose of genital stimulation. *Transvestic fetishism* is delineated as a separate category of paraphilia to refer to biological males who wear clothing of the opposite sex and, at least on some occasions, experience sexual arousal as a function of that use. These criteria must be read, however, in conjunction with the criteria set forth in the *DSM-IV-TR* (2000: xxi-xxii) for a mental disorder:

a clinically significant behavior or psychological syndrome or pattern that occurs in an individual and that is associated with present distress (e.g., a painful symptom) or disability (i.e., impairment in one or more important areas of functioning) or with a significantly increased risk of suffering death, pain, disability, or an important loss of freedom. In addition, this syndrome or pattern must not be merely an expectable and culturally sanctioned response to a particular event, for example, the death of a loved one. Whatever its original cause, it must currently be considered a manifestation of a behavioral, psychological, or biological dysfunction in the individual. Neither deviant behavior (e.g., political, religious, or sexual) nor conflicts that are primarily between the individual and society are mental disorders unless the deviance or conflict is a symptom of a dysfunction in the individual, as described above.

One must ask, then, if the behavior is not causing the individual distress or disability and does not place the individual at increased risk or suffering death, pain, disability, or an important loss of freedom, how can it be considered to be a mental disorder? How can one assess if the fantasies, urges, or behavior are causing a "clinically significant distress or impairment in social, occupational, or other important areas of functioning" absent a specification of what constitutes normative functioning in these domains? Foucault (1978), for instance, asserted that the "psychiatrization of perverse pleasure" constitutes the modern equivalent of the confessional and a form of knowledge-power. Gosselin and Wilson (1980: 23) concluded from their research:

Unusual sex patterns and predilections can be found in anyone—young or old, rich or poor, male or female. What is more, they can be found in people who otherwise don't feel themselves to be "sick" or "abnormal" in any way. It is thus doubly difficult in this field to equate "unhealthy" with "abnormal" with any degree of confidence. During our researches we came across considerable numbers of people who, while having a predilection for [fetishism, sadomasochism, or transvestism], expressed no wish to be "cured" of that predilection . . . It seems then, that no definition of abnormality in terms of "illness" is meaningful in this domain . . . .

It must be stated from the outset that, despite the research that has been conducted on fetish sexual behaviors and related sexual practices, we actually know relatively little about the behaviors that are called fetishistic and we know even less about the individuals who are attracted to and/or engage in fetishistic sexual practice, the context of those practices, the relationship between context and the fetishistic behavior, and the relationships between health effects and behavioral context. Much of the research that has been conducted to date has focused on "the acts," without examining either the nature of the relationships between the participants or the context in which they engage in sexual behavior. For instance, are individuals who utilize fetish as part of their sexual repertoire more likely to do so with steady, intimate partners or with relatively more casual partners or both? Does the level of safety that is integrated with the sexual repertoire vary depending upon the nature of the relationship (e.g., casual, long-term, steady, romantic, commercial, etc.), the setting in which the sexual behavior occurs (private residence, fetish party, group sex), the number of individuals participating, and/or the sex or other characteristics of the individuals participating? How do individuals perceive risk in the context of related behaviors, such as submission-dominance behavior and how do they address that risk? The paucity of our knowledge and our inability to respond to such basic questions ultimately limits our ability to assess associated health effects.

Fetish and Related Behaviors

What are fetish targets? Individuals may use different parts of the body (hands, feet, breasts, buttocks, armpits, and hair); clothes (handkerchiefs, stockings, underwear, corsets, and uniforms); soft materials and fabrics (fur, satin, silk, velvet, plastic, rubber, and leather); footwear (shoes and boots); and other objects (safety pins, cigarette holders, crystals, and roses, for example) by rolling in them, sucking them, burning them, cutting them, or gazing at them (Chalkley and Powell, 1983; Gosselin and Wilson, 1980). "Diaper fetishism" and "infantile fetishism," in which the individual focuses on objects symbolic of infancy such as high chairs and bibs, have been reported (Money, 1984; Pandita-Gunawardena, 1990; Malitz, 1966; Tuchman and Lachman, 1964; cf. Pate and Gabbard, 2003). The literature also contains reports of amputee fetish (Money, 1984; Wise and Kalyanam, 2000). Empirical research suggests, as well, that fetishists are particular in their interests, such as responding to particular types of shoes (sneakers, penny loafers, etc.), rather than to footwear in general (Weinberg, Williams, and Calhan, 1994).

Increasingly, fetish focus has converged on the use of specialized garments of leather and rubber (North, 1981; Steele, 1996), many of which have become integrated, to a degree, into "mainstream" fashion (Steele, 1996). Gay leather sex has been said to constitute "a celebration of Greco-Roman ideas of masculinity—a hypermale society that embraces classical male values and rituals such as honor, service, initiation, mentoring, and paying one's dues" (Brame, Brame, and Jacobs, 1993: 30).

Depending upon the nature of the relationships between the participating partners and the level of the fetishist's behavior, the partners together may engage in fetish behavior, such as one individual agreeing to wear a particular uniform or type of clothing and acting out a particular "script" that the other or both find sexually arousing. For example, a study of homosexual men with foot fetish found that many of the 262 respondents emphasized the sensual nature of the fetish object (feet and footwear), as well as its symbolic reference to masculinity (Weinberg, Williams, and Calhan, 194).

At times, fetish play may include the total coverage of the body, thereby merging fetish into a form of restriction that is equivalent to sexual bondage (Gosselin and Wilson, 1980). Similarly, a fetish attraction for particular objects and their use, such as safety pins, clips, and clamps, merges into dominance-submission behaviors/ sadomasochistic behavior. These behaviors are found in both men and women, regardless of their sexual orientation (Califia, 1983; Kamel and Weinberg, 1983).

As with fetish behavior, we actually know very little about submission-domination/sadomasochistic behavior and the context in which people engage in activities classifiable as such. We do not know, for instance, whether preferred activities vary depending upon the nature of the relationship between the participants (casual, longer-term or committed, commercial) or environmental factors; how individuals perceive these activities, choose their partners, or develop an affinity for these behaviors; the extent to which individuals perceive the possibility of injury or illness from specific practices and protect themselves from such injury; and how individuals address injury when it does occur. Although the remarks of one writer were made more than 20 years ago, they remain relevant today:

The psychiatric literature on sadomasochism is extensive. It is also relentlessly theoretical. These interrelated, often interconflicting theories have two essential features in common. All are unproven and nearly all describe and define S&M in a context of psychopathology (Mass, 1983: 49).

Accordingly, the following text provides a brief summary and description of what is known and what is believed.

The term *sadism* derives from the Marquis de Sade, a French nobleman and writer who lived during the eighteenth and nineteenth centuries. A number of his writings equate pain and humiliation with sexual pleasure (de Sade, 1976). Freud recognized the existence of some level of sadism in the "normal" individual, explaining that most men

show an admixture of aggression, of a desire to subdue, the biological significance of which lies in the necessity for overcoming the resistance of the sexual object by actions other than mere courting. Sadism would then correspond to an aggressive component of the sexual instinct which has become independent and exaggerated and has been brought to the foreground by displacement (Freud, 1938: 569).

In contrast, the term *masochism* derives from Leopold von Sacher-Masoch, who reflected his attraction to pain, humiliation, and submission in his book entitled *Venus in Furs* (1991). Krafft-Ebing (1965:86) defined masochism as

a peculiar perversion of the psychical sexual life in which the individual affected, in sexual feeling and thought, is controlled by the idea of being completely and unconditionally subject to the will of a person of the opposite sex; of being treated by this person as by a master, humiliated and abused. This idea is colored by lustful feeling; the masochist lives in fantasies, in which he creates situations of this kind and often attempts to realize them.

Clearly, this conceptualization ignores the occurrence of these behaviors between same-sex partners.

Despite this apparent distinction between those who might be sadists and those who would be masochists, Freud had posited that sadism and masochism constitute two forms of the same entity and could exist within the same individual:

He who experiences pleasure by causing pain to others in sexual relations is also capable of experiencing pain in sexual relations as pleasure. A sadist is simultaneously a masochist, though either the active or the passive side of the perversion may be more strongly developed in him and thus, represent his preponderant sexual activity (Freud, 1938: 570).

Somewhat akin to Freud's perspective, Scott (1991:ix) defined *sadomasochism* as "exchanges involving eroticized mental, emotional, or physical pain." Yet another researcher said of sadomasochism:

It is erotic, consensual, and recreational. As recreational or play-like behavior, it involves fantasy in varying degrees, which, in turn, requires some collaboration to carry out satisfactorily . . . the situation must be mutually defined by all participants as both sexual and S&M. This last idea requires that participants "frame" their behavior in certain ways by the use of social definitions that give the behavior a specific contextual meaning (Weinberg, 1987: 58).

Unlike Freud, Gebhard, an anthropologist, recognized that sadomasochism occurs within a cultural context and does not necessarily reflect psychopathology:

Sadomasochism is embedded in our culture since our culture operates on the basis of dominance-submission relationships, and aggression is socially valued. Even our gender relationships have been formulated in a structure conducive to sadomasochism: the male is supposed to be dominant and aggressive sexually and the female reluctant or submissive (Gebhard, 1969: 77).

Gebhard identified four critical features of submission-dominance behavior: the prevalence of these behaviors in literate societies, the symbolic nature of the behavior, the occurrence of the interaction between the sadist and the masochist within a social milieu, and the nature of the activity as a scripted behavior.

Sadomasochistic behavior may include, but is not limited to, restrictive, restraining, punishing, and humiliating behaviors that fall within the rubrics of bondage and discipline (B&D) and dominance and submission (D&S) (Brame, 2000; Ernulf and Innala, 1995). Sadomasochistic behavior may involve beating with hands or with instruments (paddles, whips, chains, and canes, for instance); pricking; cutting; burning; tying up; gagging; blindfolding; and immobilizing the partner, often through the use of ropes, leather devices, chains, racks, or stretchers (Hardy, 2004; Kamel, 1983; Rinella, 2004; Spectrum, 2004; Wiseman, 2004). (For an extensive listing of instruments and techniques, see Stoller, 1991.) Interaction between participants may also include various forms of verbal and mental humiliation (Gosselin and Wilson, 1980), such as mocking the partner and forcing the partner to engage in various acts, such as drinking from the toilet or allowing him- or herself to be urinated upon. Enemas may be utilized in conjunction with fetish or sadomasochistic practices (Denko, 1976).

Much of this activity, however, actually involves little pain and is centered, instead, on the idea of control, that is, of dominance and submission (Weinberg and Kamel, 1983). It has been suggested that, within the context of a relationship, as

the sexual expressions of dominance and submission, sadomasochism may be a means for some women to resolve perceived inequalities in power, perhaps in much the same way that fighting may resolve hostilities (Rian, 1982: 48).

Ethnographic research also suggests that little of this behavior is actually harmful. Stoller, a psychoanalyst, (1991: 21) concluded from his observations and interviews with S&M practitioners; managers, owners, and employees of B&D establishments; therapists; and homosexual and heterosexual pornographers that

most of the sadomasochistic acts [that he had seen and listed] are, when done by willing partners, not as bad as they seem. A Brahmin turns green watching us eat a hamburger: Whose stomach secretes the truth? When the actors know the rules and can trust their partners, there is less damage done than in many ordinary human relations, erotic or otherwise. The imitation of humiliation is carefully constructed never to produce true humiliation. The imitation of trauma, such as when being humiliated is enacted, is not traumatic. Constant, high attention to one's partner's experience is more caring and safer than the blundering, ignorant, noncommunicating obtuseness that governs so many "normal" people's erotic motions . . . We should distinguish those who harm from those who, in trying to undo the effects of harm inflicted on them early in life, play at harm. I believe it is immoral for psychoanalysts to hide their moralizing in jargon-soaked theory.

It has been suggested that "sadomasochistic behavior is best understood as a product of adult socialization processes where real or imagined sexual contact leads [individuals] to adopt new behaviors and sexual scripts" (Alison, Santtilea, Sandnabba, and Nordling, 2001: 10). Four themes have been identified within sadomasochistic scripts, with different scales of intensity within each theme. For the theme of pain, the spectrum of behaviors has been found to range from caning or the use of clothespins at one end to electrical stimulation at the other (Santtila, Sandnabba, Alison, and Nordling, 2002). For the hypermasculinity theme, rimming and watersports constitute the starting point for such activity, with the use of dildos, fistfucking, and catheters at the far extreme. The theme of humiliation includes verbal humiliation, flagellation and faceslapping as the mildest forms. The theme of restraint was reflected in behaviors with bondage at the starting point and with hypoxyphilia at the other extreme (Santtila, Sandnabba, Alison, and Nordling, 2002). Empirical research suggests that the administration and reception of pain may be more intense for gay men, while the symbolic representation of pain may be more critical for heterosexual men and women (Alison, Santtilea, Sandnabba, and Nordling, 2001). Our language may be inadequate to describe the dimensions of these experiences. As one ethnographer commented, "[T]here are not enough words for the colors of pain" (Stoller, 1991: 8).

The relatively small body of empirical research that has been conducted around sadomasochistic sexual behaviors suggests that more extreme and dangerous behavior occur relatively rarely (Spengler, 1983). Those who engage in sexual homicide may remove the victim's clothing, expose his or her genitals, position the body sexually, or perform intercourse on the victim (Myers, Burgess, Burgess, and Douglas, 1999). Lust murderers are those for whom aggression and sexuality are fused into a single experience and aggression is thereby eroticized (Myers, Burgess, Burgess, and Douglas, 1999). In these situations, the "partnering" is clearly involuntary.

Fetish behavior may also merge with *fetishistic transvestism*, apart from or in conjunction with dominance-submission/sadomasochism. Fetishistic transvestism consists only of a wish to dress in the clothing of the opposite sex, which the wearer finds sexually arousing. This form of transvestism is not indicative of either homosexuality or effeminacy (Gosselin and Wilson, 1980) and must be distinguished from *pseudotransvestism*, which involves cross-dressing without resultant sexual urges or a desire to be a member of the opposite sex, and *true transvestism*, in which the individual may assume actually consider him- or herself a member of the opposite sex (Gosselin and Wilson, 1980). Accordingly, an individual's behavior may comprise fetish, sadomasochism/submission-domination behavior and/or transvestic behavior, as illustrated below.

Origins of Fetish Practice

Numerous theories have been advanced to explain the initiation and, to a lesser extent, the maintenance of fetish behaviors. This por-

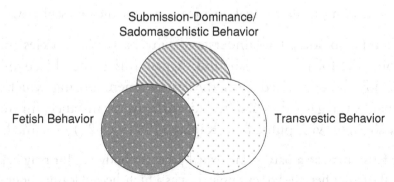

Figure 4. Relationship between Fetish Behavior, Submission-Dominance Behavior, and Transvestic Behavior

tion of the chapter provides a brief synopsis of these theories, which are variously rooted in psychoanalytic theory, biology, psychology, sociology, and anthropology. Additional references should be consulted for further examination of each of these perspectives (e.g., psychoanalytic theory: Freud, 1962; Greenacre, 1979; Nagler, 1957; sociology: Stoller, 1991; Weinberg, 1987).

Psychoanalytic Theories

Freud asserted that an adult fetishist could not overcome his aversion to female genitals without somehow endowing women with a characteristic that would make them more tolerable. Accordingly, Freud maintained, a fetish serves as protection against the threat of castration and as a token of its avoidance (Freud, 1962). Referring to Freud, Kaplan (1991: 51) has described how fetish attraction develops:

The little boy whose childhood curiosity, fantasies, anxieties, and wishes lead him to endow his mother with a substitute penis is constructing only a temporary, elusive fantasy . . . that the adult fetishist will concretize into a shoe or fur piece . . . . As Freud was the first to insist, the extravagant sexual theories of little boys may be outgrown and forgotten but they are never entirely given up. They are repressed . . . but persist as unconscious fantasies that are ready to return . . . whenever there is a serious threat, imagined or actual, to a man's hard-earned masculinity.

Freud also sought to understand why particular articles might become the focus of a fetish, and suggested that the objects might somehow be associated with the last moment during which the woman was regarded as phallic. Accordingly, for instance, fur might be associated with pubic hair. Kaplan (1991: 21-22) explained:

The fetish may be a part of the sexual partner's body . . . [or may be] the sexual partner herself. For example, just as a high-heeled leather boot may represent a female with a penis—the so-called phallic woman—so a woman, with or without boots, may be endowed with phallic properties by her fetishistic lover and thus become, for him at least, a fetish. Some fetishists are able to be sexually aroused only by policewomen or nuns or nurses, or women they command to dress up in these personalities.

More recently, researchers have both expanded on Freud's theories in order to explain the observations of fetish behavior in women (Raphling, 1987) and have formulated alternative hypotheses to explain the origin of fetishistic sexual behavior. These include evolutionary theories, theories focusing on a diseased brain as the origin of the behavior, and theories suggesting that fetishistic sexual behavior constitutes a response to a psychological experience (Wilson, 1987).

Psychoanalytic theories have also been propounded to explain the origin of behaviors that are sometimes related to fetishism, such as sadism and masochism. Shainess (1997: 552) has argued both that masochism constitutes a "serious character-personality warp" and that masochists actually fear and hate others and hold them in contempt. Shainess further asserts that masochism is more common in women than in men due to social reinforcement.

Biological Theories

A number of researchers have argued that fetish behavior has a biological basis. Epstein (1960) has asserted, for instance, that characteristics of fetishism approximate temporal lobe dysfunction. Mitchell and colleagues (1954) described an individual with a safety pin fetish, whose fetish disappeared following a temporal lobectomy designed to address his temporal lobe epilepsy. Yet another case report focused on an individual whose fetish appeared following the onset of a temporal lobe tumor (Ball, 1968). Case reports have described the development of a foot fetish following the onset of multiple sclerosis (Huws, Shubsachs, and Taylor, 1991) and of fetishism subsequent to suffering traumatic head injury with generalized abnormalities indicated on an electroencephalogram (Pandita-Gunawardena, 1990). Case reports are, however, inadequate to establish a causal link.

Psychological Theories

A number of researchers have hypothesized that, based on classical conditioning theory, individuals' sexual response system becomes conditioned to respond to particular stimuli that are characteristics of the potential sexual partner, such as feet, shoes, etc. and consequently becomes preoccupied sexually with that stimulus rather than the partner associated with it. Empirical research has demonstrated, for instance, that men may be conditioned under experimental conditions to develop an erection in response to specific stimuli, such as boots (Rachman, 1966; Rachman and Hodgson, 1968). Reinforcement to maintain the behavior over an extended period of time may result from masturbation and orgasm (McGuire, Carlisle, and Young, 1965). Other researchers, however, have criticized the reliance on classical conditioning theory to explain fetish behavior, arguing that it fails to explain why some individuals develop fetishism and others do not (Wilson, 1987).

Social learning theory has also been utilized to explain the development of fetish behavior. Gebhardt (1969) postulated that young males, such as adolescents, are particularly susceptible to the association of sex with symbols, which are encountered prior to experiencing sociosexual gratification. La Torre (1980) demonstrated experimentally that men who believe themselves to have been rejected by a woman are more likely than men who believe themselves to be accepted to rate garments and body parts of a woman as more attractive than the whole woman. These findings raise questions regarding the link between levels of self-esteem, previous experiences, perceived inadequacy, and fetish behavior.

Sociobiological and Sociocultural Factors

It has been asserted that fetish behavior may be subject to the influence of cultural factors (Wise, 1985). As an example, the previous Chinese practice of binding women's feet is considered to be a fetish. Foot binding is believed to have begun during the Southern Sung Dynasty (1127-1279 A.D.). The practice, which began with palace dancers, involved compression of the foot, resulting in a distorted foot with a swollen ankle and a need to rely on a cane for support (Breiner, 1992). In silhouette, the foot assumed the appearance of a high-heeled shoe (Steele, 1996). The bound female foot, referred to as "Lotus," was a component of foreplay, which often included kissing, sucking, nibbling and pressing the foot against the male genitals. Foot binding was not, however,

one monolithic, unchanging experience that all unfortunate women in each succeeding dynasty went through, but is rather an amorphous practice that meant different things to different people . . . It is, in other words, a situated practice (Ko, 1994).

The later prohibition of foot binding was premised on the rude and overtly sexual nature of the practice (Breiner, 1992).

Theories of Differences

It is believed that fetishism occurs more frequently in men than in women (Mason, 1997). Transvestic fetishism in women has been said to be "so rare it is almost nonexistent" (Stoller, 1982). However, due to the relative scarcity of studies focusing on the prevalence of fetishism and the relative rarity with which individuals engaged in fetish practice present for clinical practice, it is impossible to say how much more frequently men than women engage in fetishism (Mason, 1997). Several theories have been developed to explain why men might more frequently engage in fetish behavior.

Kinsey and colleagues (1953), who observed few women with fetishism, postulated that fetish attraction or behavior occurs more frequently in men because men are conditioned more easily by their sexual experiences and by objects that are associated with those experiences. Gosselin and Wilson (1980) also speculated that men might be more likely to be fetishists due to the visual nature of fetishism, men's sensitivity to visual stimuli, and the biofeedback provided by the penis. Other researchers have focused on understanding the lower incidence of fetishism among women and have variously postulated that it may result from the protective effect against "abnormal" stimuli that is afforded women by the lack of a clear genital signal (an erect penis) (Bancroft, 1989) or women's need to identify an appropriate sexual partner as efficiently as possible due to a limited number of eggs (Wilson, 1987). The effects of prenatal hormones have also been offered as a possible explanation for the difference in fetish frequency between men and women (Pitcher, 1990).

Researchers have noted the common assumption that gay men are more likely to engage in sadomasochistic sexual behaviors than either heterosexual men or women, fewer women than men engage in sadomasochistic behaviors, and that those who do are most likely to be prostitutes (Breslow, Evans, and Langley, 1985; Levitt, Moser, and Jamison, 1994). The relatively few research studies that have been conducted with women indicate that women who are not engaged in commercial sex work who do engage in sadomasochistic sexual encounters tend to be better educated than the general population, and are also less likely to be married (Levitt, Moser, and Jamison, 1994). The behavior is not exclusive to a particular sexual orientation, and can be found among women who self-identify as heterosexual, bisexual, and lesbian (Levitt, Moser, and Jamison, 1994).

Fetish and Health

Relatively little research has been conducted relating to the health effects of fetish or related practices, such as submission-dominance behaviors and sadomasochistic practices. Even less research has examined the partnering in which these behaviors occur or the longitudinal effects of these partnerings and the contexts in which they occur. The following represents a brief summary of the research that exists to date, with recommendations for further research and clinical practice.

Physical Violence

Prior research indicates that there may exist four primary points during which an individual engaging in S&M activities must pay particular attention to the possibility of physical violence: the locations that facilitate S&M encounters, such as clubs and bars; the screening of partners; the negotiation of the scenario that is to occur; and the control of interaction during scenario (Lee, 1983).

In the gay S&M scene, encounters are often facilitated through leather bars, leather clubs, and leather baths. The costume that is expected at these locations may serve as a mechanism for controlling entry. Standardized colors and signals, such as the placement of a handkerchief or scarf of a particular color, provide potential sexual partners with preliminary information regarding an individual's preferred activities (Lee, 1983; Wiseman, 1996). The actual screening of a potential partner, however, is left to the individual. Oftentimes, because there are often a limited number of establishments catering to S&M-interested individuals, the proposed partner may be a familiar face in the bar or may have earned a reputation to other bar clientele or to the bartender. Although there exists a danger of encountering a real sadist, there is a greater like-lihood of encountering danger and risk at the hands of an individual who becomes engulfed in playing role (Lee, 1983)

Risks that have been identified in conjunction with gay S&M sex include being detained longer than desired, more uncomfortable positions or conditions than desired, being subjected to more discipline than desired, and actual physical torture. A study of 35 gay men in Toronto who participated in S&M behaviors over 3 year period identified various problems, including beating that went beyond the point of pleasant endurance; agreed upon bondage during which several friends of the master engaged in anal sex with the "slave" without his prior agreement; bondage until feeling was lost in limbs; and an accident involving a piece of equipment (Lee, 1983). A total of 11 out of "several hundred" incidents, consisting of reports by 9 of 35 men, resulted in physical harm requiring medical treatment (Lee, 1983). The total number of incidents remained unspecified by the author.

Empirical research indicates that many heterosexual individuals who engage in fetish or submission-dominance behavior locate and access prospective partners through websites, subculture publications, organizations, parties, and specialized clubs (Becker, 1963; Gagnon, 1977; Smith and Cox, 1979; Weinberg, 1978; Weinberg, Williams, and Calhan, 1994). Consumer-oriented publications provide information on how to place and answer personal ads for partners and how to find partners at clubs, through organizations, and through cyberspace (e.g., Wiseman, 1996). Prostitution appears to be an especially important source of partners and contacts for heterosexual men (DeLora and Warren, 1977; Halpern, 1977; Spengler, 1977). Although heterosexual cruising baths exist, the relatively little research that has been conducted with regards to this milieu suggests that, unlike some of the gay clubs and baths, "no etiquette of public sex" exists (Lee, 1983: 177), potentially increasing the risk of physical violence.

An increasing consumer-oriented literature has become available to provide risk-reduction advice to individuals engaging in S&M sex. One author has bluntly stated, "S&M is the riskiest form of sex. Even under ideal conditions, with all & reasonable precautions taken, danger sometimes appears" (Wiseman, 1996). Much of this advice centers on avoiding a "session" while under the influence of alcohol or other substances (Wiseman, 1996); avoiding the use of inappropriate or worn-out equipment (Wiseman, 1996); disregarding safewords or failing to agree upon safewords ahead of time to end a particular activity (Henkin and Holiday, 1996; Wiseman, 1996; Wiseman, 2004); the need to know appropriate first aid and CPR measures should an emergency occur (Wiseman, 1996; Wiseman, 2004), and precautions to be taken in conjunction with specific activities or pieces of equipment (e.g., Henkin and Holiday, 1996).

Discussions within S&M communities have focused, as well, on the need to distinguish between S&M sex and partner abuse. Some groups, such as the National Leather Association, provide information to their members and encourage them to recognize when they are being abused, to report the abuse, and to seek assistance (Brame, 2000).

Mental Health

Almost no research has been conducted on the short-term or long-term health effects of engaging in fetish or related behaviors with sexual partners. One researcher has noted the possibility that casual sex may lead to feelings of ego bruising rejection (Lee, 1983). However, sex may be casual regardless of the nature of the sexual activity. Henkin and Holiday (1996), recognizing the difference between the therapeutic potential of any event or experience, regardless of its nature, and the therapeutic process, have advised their readers to avoid "doing psychotherapy in the dungeon" in an attempt to resolve past issues.

Sexually Transmitted Disease

A number of consumer-oriented publications provide advice regarding strategies to avoid the transmission of sexually transmitted infections (e.g., Wiseman, 1996). To date, however, there appears to be no empirical research that has focused on individuals' perception of risk in the context of fetish/S&M behaviors; how conceptualizations of risk relate to strategies for the screening and selection of partners; and how the context or environment in which the sexual activity occurs mediates the level of risk or protection that is perceived and/or accepted by the participants.

Implications for Research and Practice

References

Alison, L., Santtila, P., Sandnabba, N.K., Nordling, N. (2001). Sadomasochistically oriented behavior: Diversity in practice and meaning. *Archives of Sexual Behavior* 30(1): 1-12.

American Psychiatric Association. (2000). *Diagnostic and Statistical Manual of Mental Disorders, Fourth Edition, Text Revision (DSM-IV-TR)*. Washington, D.C.: American Psychiatric Association.

Balachandra, K. (2002). Fire fetishism in a female arsonist? *Canadian Journal of Psychiatry* 47(5): 487-488.

Ball, J.R.B. (1968). A case of hair fetishism, transvestism, and organic cerebral disorder. *Acta Psychiatrica Scandinavia* 44: 249-254.

Bancroft, J. (1989). *Human Sexuality and Its Problems*, 2nd ed. Edinburgh: Churchill Livingstone.

Becker, H.S. (1963). *Outsiders: Studies in the Sociology of Deviance*. New York: Free Press.

Brame, G.G. (2000). *Come Hither: A Commonsense Guide to Kinky Sex*. New York: Simon & Schuster.

Brame, G.G., Brame, W.D., Jacobs, J. (1993). *Different Loving: The World of Sexual Dominance and Submission*. New York: Villard.

Breiner, S.J. (1992). Sexuality in traditional China: Its relationship to child abuse. *Child Psychiatry and Human Development* 23(2): 53-67.

Breslow, N., Evans, L., Langley, J. (1985). On the prevalence and roles of females in the sadomasochistic subculture: Report of an empirical study. *Archives of Sexual Behavior* 14(4): 303-317.

Califia, P. (1983). A secret side of lesbian sexuality. In T. Weinberg, G.W.L. Kamel (Eds.), *S and M: Studies in Sadomasochism* (pp. 129-136). Buffalo, New York: Prometheus Books.

Chalkley, A.J., Powell, G.E. (1983). The clinical description of forty-eight cases of sexual fetishism. *British Journal of Psychiatry* 142: 292-295.

De Sade, Marquis. (1976, trans.). *The 120 Days of Sodom and Other Writings* (A. Wainhouse, Trans.). New York: Grove/Atlantic, Inc.

DeLora, J.S., Warren, C.A.B. (1977). *Understanding Sexual Interaction.* Boston: Houghton-Mifflin.

Denko, J.D. (1976). Klismaphilia: Amplification of the erotic enema device. *American Journal of Psychotherapy* 30(2): 236-255.

Enulf, K.E., Innala, S.M. (1995). Sexual bondage: A review and unobtrusive investigation. *Archives of Sexual Behavior* 24(6): 631-654.

Epstein, A.W. (1960). Fetishism: A study of its psychopathology with particular reference to a proposed disorder in brain mechanisms as an etiologic factor. *Journal of Nervous and Mental Disorders* 130: 107-119.

Foucault, M. (1978). *The History of Sexuality*, vol. 1: *An Introduction.* (R. Hurley, trans.). New York: Random House.

Freud, S. (1938). *The Basic Writings of Sigmund Freud.* (A.A. Brill, trans. and ed.). New York: Modern Library.

Freud, S. Fetishism. In *The Standard Edition of the Complete Psychological Work*, vol. 1. London: Hogarth Press and The Institute for Psychoanalysis, 1953-1975.

Freud, S. (1962). Three essays on theories of sexuality. In J. Strachey (Ed., Trans.), *The Standard Edition of the Complete Psychological Works of Sigmund Freud* (vol. 7). London: Hogarth Press. (original work published 1905).

Gagnon, J. (1977). *Human Sexualities.* Glenview, Illinois: Scott, Foresman.

Gamman, L. Makinen, M. (1994). *Female Fetishism: A New Look*. London: Lawrence & Wishart.

Gebhardt, P. (1969). Fetishism and sado-masochism. *Science and Psychoanalysis* 15: 71-80.

Gebhardt, P.H. (1969). Fetishism and sadomasochism. In J.H. Masserman (Ed.). *Dynamics of Deviant Sexuality* (pp. 71-80). New York: Grune & Stratton.

Gosselin, C., Wilson, G. (1980). *Sexual Variations: Fetishism, Sadomasochism, Transvestism*. London: Faber & Faber.

Greenacre, P. (1979). Fetishism. In I. Rosen (Ed.), *Sexual Deviation*. Oxford, England: Oxford University Press.

Halpern, B. (1977). Spanks for the memory. *Screw* 420 (March 21): 4-7.

Hardy, J.W. (2004). *Canes and Caning*. Oakland, California: Greenery Press.

Henkin, W.A., Holiday, S.(1996). *Consensual Sadomasochism: How to Talk About It & How to Do It Safely*. Los Angeles, California: Daedalus Publishing Company.

Huws, R., Shubsachs, A.P.W., Taylor, P.J. (1991). Hypersexuality, fetishism, and multiple sclerosis. *British Journal of Psychiatry* 158: 280-281.

Kamel, G.W.L. (1983). Leathersex: Meaningful aspects of gay sado-masochism. In T. Weinberg, G.W.L. Kamel (Eds.), *S and M: Studies in Sadomasochism* (pp. 162-174). Buffalo, New York: Prometheus Books.

Kamel, G.W.L., Weinberg, T.S. (1983). Diversity in sadomasochism: Four S&M careers. In T. Weinberg, G.W.L. Kamel (Eds.), *S and M: Studies in Sadomasochism* (pp. 113-128). Buffalo, New York: Prometheus Books.

Kaplan, L. (1991). *Female Perversions: The Temptations of Emma Bovary*. New York: Doubleday.

Kinsey, A.C., Pomeroy, W.B., Martin, C.E., Gebhard, P.H. (1953). *Sexual Behavior in the Human Female*. New York: Simon & Schuster.

Ko, D. (1994). Talking about footbinding: Discourses of manhood and nationhood in Late Imperial China. Paper delivered at panel, The Mindful Body: Footbinding, Forty-Sixth Annual Meeting of the Association for Asian Studies, March 26. Quoted in V. Steele (1996).

Fetish: Fashion, Sex & Power (p. 93). New York: Oxford University Press.

Krafft-Ebing, R. von. (1965). *Psychopathia Sexualis* (F.S. Klaf, trans.). New York: Stein and Day.

Krafft-Ebing, R. von. (1886). *Psychopathia Sexualis with Especial Reference to the Antipathic Sexual Instinct: A Medico-Forensic Study* (F.J. Rebman, trans.). New York: Physicians and Surgeons Book Company, 1906, 1934.

La Torre, R. (1980). Devaluation of the human love object: Heterosexual rejection as a possible antecedent of fetishism. *Journal of Abnormal Psychology* 89: 295-298.

Lee, J.A. (1983). The social organization of sexual risk. In T. Weinberg, G.W.L. Kamel (Eds.), *S and M: Studies in Sadomasochism* (pp. 175-193). Buffalo, New York: Prometheus Books.

Levitt, E.E., Moser, C., Jamison, K.V. (1994). The prevalence and some attributes of females in the sadomasochistic subculture: A second report. *Archives of Sexual Behavior* 23(4): 465-473.

Malitz, S. (1966). Another report on the wearing of diapers and rubber pants by an adult male. *American Journal of Psychiatry* 122: 1435-1437.

Mason, F.L. (1997). Fetishism: Psychopathology and theory. In D.R. Lewis, W. O'Donohue (Eds.), *Sexual Deviance: Theory, Assessment, and Treatment* (pp. 75-91). New York: Guilford Press.

Mass, L. (1983), Coming to grips with sadomasochism. In T. Weinberg, G.W.L. Kamel (Eds.), *S and M: Studies in Sadomasochism* (pp. 45-56). Buffalo, New York: Prometheus Books.

McGuire, R.J., Carlisle, J.M., Young, B.G. (1965). Sexual deviations as conditioned behaviour: A hypothesis. *Behaviour Research and Therapy* 2: 185-190.

Mitchell, W., Falconer, M.A., Hill, D. (1954). Epilepsy with fetishism relieved by temporal lobectomy. *Lancet* 2: 626-630.

Money, J. (1984). Paraphilias: Phenomenology and classification. *American Journal of Psychotherapy* 38(2): 164-179.

Myers, W.C., Burgess, A.W., Burgess, A.G., Douglas, J.E. (1999). Serial murder and sexual homicide. In V. Van Hasselt, M. Hersen (Eds.),

Handbook of Psychological Approaches with Violent Offenders (pp. 153-172). New York: Kluwer Academic/Plenum Publishers.

Nagler, S.H. (1957). Fetishism: A review and case study. *Psychiatric Quarterly* 10: 713-770.

North, M. (1981). *The Outer Fringe of Sex: A Study in Sexual Fetishism.* London: Odyssey Press.

Pandita-Gunawardena, R. (1990). Paraphilia infantilism: A rare case of fetishistic behaviour. *British Journal of Psychiatry* 157: 767-770.

Pate, J.E., Gabbard, G.O. (2003). Adult baby syndrome. *American Journal of Psychiatry* 160(11): 1932-1936.

Pitcher, D. (1990). Fetishism. In R. Bluglass, P. Bowden (Eds.), *Principles and Practice of Forensic Psychiatry.* Edinburgh: Churchill Livingstone.

Rachman, S. (1966). Sexual fetishism: An experimental analogue. *Psychological Record* 16: 293-296.

Rachman, S., Hodgson, R. (1968). Experimentally induced "sexual fetishism": Replication and development. *Psychological Record* 18: 25-27.

Raphling, D.L. (1989). Fetishism in a woman. *Journal of the American Psychoanalytic Association* 37: 465-491.

Rian, K. (1982). S/M and the social construction of desire. In R.R. Linden, D.R. Pagano, D.E.H. Russell, S.L. Star (Eds.). *Against Sadomasochism: A Radical Feminist Analysis* (pp. 45-49). San Francisco, California: Frog in the Wall.

Richards, A.K. (1990). Female fetishes and female perversions: Hermine Hug-Hellmuth's "A Case of Female Foot or More Properly Boot Fetishism" reconsidered. *Psychoanalytic Review* 77(1): 11-23.

Rinella, J. (2004). *Clips and Clamps.* Oakland, California: Greenery Press.

Von Sacher-Masoch, L. (1991). *Venus in Furs.* In J. McNeil (Trans.), *Masochism* (pp. 143-271). New York: Zone Books.

Santtila, P., Sandnabba, N.K., Alison, L., Nordling, N. (2002). Investigating the underlying structure in sadomasochistically oriented behavior. *Archives of Sexual Behavior* 31(2): 185-196.

Scott, G.G. (1991). *Erotic Power: An Exploration of Dominance and Submission.* New York: Citadel Press.

Shainess, N. (1997). Masochism revisited: Reflections on masochism and its childhood antecedents. *American Journal of Psychotherapy* 51(4): 552-568.

Smith, H., Cox, C. (1979). Scenes: s&m in the open. *Village Voice* 24 (Jan. 15): 24.

Spectrum. (2004). *Hot Wax and Temperature Play*. Oakland, California: Greenery Press.

Spengler, A. (1983). Manifest sadomasochism of males: Results of an empirical study. In T. Weinberg, G.W.L. Kamel (Eds.), *S and M: Studies in Sadomasochism* (pp. 57-72). Buffalo, New York: Prometheus Books.

Steele, V. (1996). *Fetish: Fashion, Sex & Power*. New York: Oxford University Press.

Stoller, R.J. (1991). *Pain and Passion: A Psychoanalyst Explores the World of S&M*. New York: Plenum Press.

Stoller, R.J. (1982). Transvestism in women. *Archives of Sexual Behavior* 11(2): 99-115.

Tuchman, W.W., Lachman, J.H. (1964). An unusual perversion: The wearing of diapers and rubber pants in a 29 year old male. *American Journal of Psychiatry* 120: 1198-1199.

Webster's Third New International Dictionary Unabridged (1986).

Weinberg, M.S., Williams, C.J., Calhan, C. (1994). Homosexual foot fetishism. *Archives of Sexual Behavior* 23(6): 611-626.

Weinberg, T.S. (1978). Sadism and masochism: Sociological perspectives. *Bulletin of the American Academy of Psychiatry and the Law* 6: 284-295.

Weinberg, T.S. (1987). Sadomasochism in the United States: A review of recent sociological literature. *The Journal of Sex Research* 23(1): 50-69.

Weinberg, T.S., Kamel, G.W.L. (1983). S&M: An introduction to the study of sadomasochism. In T. Weinberg, G.W.L. Kamel (Eds.), *S and M: Studies in Sadomasochism* (pp. 17-24). Buffalo, New York: Prometheus Books.

Wilson, G. (1987). An ethological approach to sexual deviation. In G. Wilson (Ed.), *Variant Sexuality: Research and Theory*. London: Croon Helm.

Wilson, G. (1987). *Variant Sexuality: Research and Theory*. Baltimore, Maryland: Johns Hopkins Press.

Wise, T.N. (1985). Fetishism: Etiology and treatment. A review from multiple perspectives. *Comprehensive Psychiatry* 26(3): 249-257.

Wise, T.N., Kalyanam, R.C. (2000). Amputee fetishism and genital mutilation: Case report and literature review. *Journal of Sex & Marital Therapy* 26: 339-344.

Wiseman, J. (2004). *Dungeon Emergencies and Supplies*. Oakland, California: Greenery Press.

Wiseman, J. (1996). *SM101: A Realistic Introduction*. San Francisco, California: Greenery Press.

CHAPTER 6

Conclusion

As suggested in the Prologue, the data that are presented in this text are not new. However, it is hoped that their integration into one volume concerned with sexual partnering, sexual practices, and health will instigate thoughtful discussion about their underlying commonalities and the possibilities for furthering our knowledge with respect to each of the topics discussed.

What is strikingly clear from this review is our lack of language that can encompass the multiple dimensions and infinite nuances inherent in partnerings. We can visualize the multiple axes across which relationships are constructed, including the legal, religious, and moral. Concepts of pedophilia, incest, and child molestations have been so conflated that it often becomes difficult to distinguish exactly what the focus of a discussion, study or policy actually is. Concepts of commercial sex work, trafficking, and immigration overlap; these terms are used by multiple writers, researchers, and policymakers in the mistaken belief that they are referring to the same set of circumstances. Our lack of language to define our experiences has implications not only for our ability to communicate across disciplines but also for our ability to examine and address the health issues that arise in and from partnering situations and the environments in which they occur. As one writer commented,

The power of naming is at least two-fold, naming defines the quality and value of that which is named—and it also denies reality and value to that which is never named, never uttered. That which has no name, that for which we have no words or concepts, is rendered mute and invisible; powerless to inform or transform our consciousness of our experience, our understanding, our vision, powerless to claim its own existence (DuBois, 1983: 198).

What is equally clear is that we are frighteningly ignorant of the many of the details that characterize the contexts in which the partnerings occur and the health implications of their occurrence. To a large extent, it would appear that our ignorance stems not from our inability to learn about these contexts, but rather from an unwillingness to do so and a reticence—or is it fear?—that allows us, instead, to continue to rest on untested and unverified assumptions.

As an example of these assumptions, consider the following tautologies that appear to pervade our cultural psyche:

Monogamy is good.
Monogamy is marriage.
You can only be married to one person.
Those who are in nonmonogamous relationships are immoral.

Commercial sex work is immoral.
No one would engage in commercial sex work willingly.
If someone engages in commercial sex work, they must have been forced to do so.
If they were not forced into commercial sex work, they must be flawed as the result of incest or child abuse.

Pain is bad.
Pain is to be avoided at all costs.
If someone does something to another person that would cause me pain, it must also cause the other person pain.
If they are causing the other person pain, it must be abuse.
If it is abuse, it must be punished.
If it is not causing the other person pain, and they are enjoying it, there must be something wrong with them.

Ultimately, those who resist compliance with these cultural edicts or who seemingly, intentionally or not, appear to fall outside the boundaries that they establish, are regarded as flawed or deviant for having violated these norms (Black, 1976; Clinard and Meier, 1979; Davis, 1975; Feldman, 1978). Unfortunately, all too often, these cultural assumptions are transformed into political agendas and policy determinations without appropriate investigation and research and without an adequate understanding of relevant individual, partner-level, family-level, institutional level, and systemic factors and their interplay. Consider, again, the following.

- We proclaim the superiority of the two-parent household as a mechanism for healthy child development and reduction of risk of sexually transmitted infections between the partners, without regard to the quality of that exchange, the existence or quality of other relationships that comprise the family network, and without adequate research to substantiate that proclamation.

- We prohibit, for the most part, commercial sex work where the partnering is premised on an exchange of sexual favors for currency between the individual participating in the sex act, but permit the same activity in exchange for payment by a third party, such as an adult film producer. We lament incessantly the potential for transmission of sexually transmitted diseases as a result of commercial sex work, which is perceived as a public health problem, but conveniently overlook data that appear to indicate that rates of violence against commercial sex workers rose in many U.S. venues following the eradication of red light districts. We know little about why individuals choose to engage as sex workers; how they formulate the decision to do so; how they perceive their health and health risks; and if, when, and how they extricate themselves from commercial sex work, although these issues may be critical to the prevention of disease and the creation of effective interventions. We know even less about why "johns" engage the services of commercial sex workers and the factors and contexts that encourage or discourage their demands for these services, despite the fact that the "johns," in many ways, are similarly situated in terms of potential health concerns.

- Despite the increased law enforcement efforts and media attention focused on trafficking, we have relatively little information about the historical, geographical, socioeconomic, cultural, and political circumstances that create an environment in which trafficking can occur, the factors that propel individuals to engage as traffickers, and the various circumstances in which individuals become trafficked. Our refusal to acknowledge and address the reality that some individuals may voluntarily choose to be trafficked and/or engage in commercial sex work hampers not only law enforcement efforts, which appear to be the primary concern of many national laws and international discourse, but also our ability to understand when and how to best provide health care assistance.

Ultimately, we must evaluate how we know what we know and if that knowledge is "real." A failure or refusal to examine multiple facets of partnerings and the contexts in which they occur preordains an inability to address adequately the health needs of patients, clients, and communities. Consider, as but one concrete example, the history of our efforts to reduce HIV transmission.

In 1981, *Pneumocystis carinii* pneumonia (PCP) was reported in five homosexual men (Centers for Disease Control, 1981a) and Kaposi's sarcoma was identified in 26 others (Centers for Disease Control, 1981b). Ultimately, both conclusions were linked to an underlying immune deficiency (Gottlieb et al., 1981; Masur et al., 1981). The illness, initially known as gay-related immune deficiency (Gottlieb et al., 1982), was attributed to lifestyle choices: "the fact that these patients were all homosexuals suggests an association between some aspect of homosexual lifestyle or disease acquired through sexual contact and *Pneumocystis* pneumonia in this population" (Centers for Disease Control, 1986: 2). The ailment was later noted among Haitians, hemophiliacs, and injection drug users (Shilts, 1987), prompting the identification of groups at risk for contracting HIV/AIDS: homosexuals, heroin users, Haitians, and hemophiliacs (New York City Commission on

Human Rights, 1986, 1987). On March 4, 1983, the Centers for Disease Control specifically referred to high-risk groups, defining them as groups whose members were both at higher risks of contacting HIV infection and of infecting others (Oppenheimer, 1992).

Those individuals identified as gay, bisexual, or intravenous drug users would henceforth be identified as a member of a group with an increased risk of HIV infection, regardless of whether the individual actually engaged in behavior that was linked to an increased risk of HIV transmission. AIDS risk groups were depicted as somehow culturally different as well as deviant. Diversity within groups was ignored and stereotyping became common (Schiller, Crystal, and Lewellen, 1994). Such stereotyping carries serious implications for HIV prevention, diagnosis, and care.

For example, homosexuals were perceived as harbingers of disease (New York City Commission on Human Rights, 1986, 1987; Wyatt, 1991). The culture of gay men was depicted as involving multiple sexual partners, frequent sexual activity in bath houses, use of sex-enhancing drugs, oral-genital contact, and anal intercourse, without regard to the variations in frequency and manner of sexual activity among gay men (Schiller et al., 1994). Such generalizations carry serious implications for these individuals. First, negatively stereotyped patients might receive less than adequate care (Najman, Klein, and Munro, 1982), or may be viewed by their providers as more responsible for and deserving of their illness and less deserving of sympathy than other patients (Kelly et al., 1987). Second, an emphasis on homosexuality, rather than on unprotected sexual intercourse between men, results in the exclusion and self-exclusion of men who have sex with men but who do not self-identify as either homosexual or bisexual due to political, cultural, or other connotations (Jonsen and Stryker, 1993).

Additionally, the initial construction of AIDS based on symptoms and manifestations noted in men adversely affected women's care in a number of ways. Prior to the 1993 revision of the AIDS case definition (Centers for Disease Control, 1992), defining criteria for an AIDS diagnosis included PCP, toxoplasmosis, Kaposi's sarcoma and other cancers, oral candidiasis, and wasting (Institute of Medicine, 1988). These criteria did not include numerous other conditions that were noted among HIV-infected women, including cervical cancer, pelvic inflammatory disease, human papillomavirus, recurrent or persistent herpes simplex virus, and recurrent or persistent genital candidiasis (American Public Health Association, 1991; Anastos and Marte, 1989). Cervical dysplasia, which is more than eight times likely to occur in HIV-infected women than in noninfected women (American Public Health Association, 1991), was similarly omitted as a diagnostic criterion until 1993 (Centers for Disease Control, 1992), 12 years after the initial identification of the disease. This omission of conditions affecting HIV-infected women from the AIDS case definition resulted in the underdiagnosis of AIDS among women and the inability of many women to qualify for publicly funded benefits such as Medicare and disability (American Public Health Association, 1991; Roper and Winkenwerder, 1988), and may have contributed to differential survival times among women due to lack of access to appropriate care (American Public Health Association, 1991).

While some might argue that more recent research findings challenge the previously existing generalizations and stereotypes of HIV and permitted the dissipation of such views, it is also likely that such research was regarded as unnecessary and superfluous precisely because of underlying assumptions and generalizations regarding susceptibility to infection. This example underscores the critical importance of engaging in a continuous evaluation of our knowledge and how we think we know what we think we know.

References

American Public Health Association. (1991). *Women and HIV Disease: A Report of the Special Initiative on AIDS of the American Public Health Association.* Washington, D.C.: American Public Health Association.

Anastos, K., Marte, C. (1989). The missing persons in the AIDS epidemic. Health PAC Bulletin. Cited in S.C. Quinn. (1993). AIDS and the African American woman: The triple burden of race, class, and gender. *Health Education Quarterly* 20: 305-320.

Black, D. (1976). *The Behavior of Law.* New York: Academic Press.

Centers for Disease Control. (1981a). Pneumocystis pneumonia—Los Angeles. *Morbidity and Mortality Weekly Report* 30: 250-252.

Centers for Disease Control. (1981b). Kaposi's sarcoma and Pneumocystis pneumonia among homosexual men—New York City and California. *Morbidity and Mortality Weekly Report* 30: 305-308.

Centers for Disease Control. (1986). *Reports on AIDS Published in the Morbidity and Mortality Weekly Report, June 1981 through February 1986.* Springfield, Virginia: National technical Information Service.

Centers for Disease Control. (1992). 1993 revised classification system for HIV infection and expanded surveillance case definition for AIDS among adolescents and adults. *Morbidity and Mortality Weekly Report* 41, No. RR-17.

Clinard, M.B., Meier, R.F. (1979). *The Sociology of Deviant Behavior,* 5th ed. New York: Holt, Rinehart, and Winston.

Davis, N.J. (1975). *The Social Construction of Deviance.* Dubuque, Iowa: William C. Brown.

Du Bois, B. (1983). Passionate scholarship: Notes on values, knowing and method in feminist social science. In G. Bowles, R.D. Klein (Eds.), *Theories of Women's Studies.* London: Routledge & Kegan Paul.

Feldman, S.D., (Ed.). (1978). *Deciphering Deviance.* Boston: Little Brown.

Gottlieb, M.S., Schroff, R., Fligiel, S., Fahey, J.L., Saxon, A. (1982). Gay-related immunodeficiency (GRID) syndrome: Clinical and autopsy observations. *Clinical Research* 30: 349A.

Gottlieb, M.S., Schroff, R., Schanker, H.M., Weisman, J.D., Peng, T.F.A, Wolf, R.A., Saxon, A. (1981). *Pneumocystis carinii* pneumonia ad mucosal candidiasis in previously healthy homosexual men: Evidence of a newly acquired immunodeficiency. *New England Journal of Medicine* 305: 1425-1431.

Jonsen, A.R., Stryker, J. (Eds.). (1993). *The Social Impact of AIDS in the United States.* Washington, D.C.: National Academy Press.

Kelly, J.A., St. Lawrence, J.T., Smith, S., Hood, H.V., Cook, D.J. (1987). Stigmatization of AIDS patients by physicians. *American Journal of Public Health* 77: 789-791.

Najman, J.M., Klein, D., Munro, C. (1982). Patient characteristics negatively stereotyped by doctors. *Social Science and Medicine* 16: 1781-1789.

New York City Commission on Human Rights. (1986, November). *AIDS and People of Color: The Discriminatory Impact.* New York: Author.

New York City Commission on Human Rights. (1987, August). *AIDS Discrimination and Its Implications for People of Color and Other Minorities.* New York: Author.

Oppenheimer, G.M. (1992). Causes, cases, and cohorts: The role of epidemiology in the historical construction of AIDS. In E. Fee, D.M. Fox (Eds.), *AIDS: The Making of a Chronic Disease* (pp. 49-83). Berkeley, California: University of California Press.

Schiller, N.G., Crystal, S., Lewellen, D. (1994). Risky business: The cultural construction of AIDS risk groups. *Social Science and Medicine* 38: 1337-1346.

Shilts, R. (1987). *And the Band Played On: Politics, People, and the AIDS Epidemic.* New York: St. Martin's Press.

Index